I HATE Myself NOW WHAT?

I HATE Myself NOW WHAT?

A Step-by-Step Workbook for You and Your Therapist

Blaise Aguirre, MD

WILEY

Published by John Wiley & Sons, Inc., Hoboken, New Jersey.

For general information on our other products and services or for technical support, please contact our Customer Care Department within the United States at (800) 762-2974, outside the United States at (317) 572-3993 or fax (317) 572-4002.

Wiley also publishes its books in a variety of electronic formats. Some content that appears in print may not be available in electronic formats. For more information about Wiley products, visit our web site at www.wiley.com.

Library of Congress Cataloging-in-Publication Data:

Names: Aguirre, Blaise, 1964- author
Title: I hate myself. Now what? : A step-by-step workbook for you and your therapist / Blaise Aguirre.
Description: Hoboken, New Jersey : Wiley, [2026] | Includes index.
Identifiers: LCCN 2025054685 (print) | LCCN 2025054686 (ebook) | ISBN 9781394389759 paperback | ISBN 9781394389773 adobe pdf | ISBN 9781394389766 epub
Subjects: LCSH: Self-hate (Psychology)
Classification: LCC BF697.5.S429 A483 2026 (print) | LCC BF697.5.S429 (ebook)
LC record available at https://lccn.loc.gov/2025054685
LC ebook record available at https://lccn.loc.gov/2025054686

Cover Design: Wiley
Cover Images: © Douglas Baldan/Shutterstock, © klyaksun/Shutterstock

SKY10149026_030626

To everyone who has faced the often-silent battle of self-hatred and yet found the courage to seek a deeper understanding, dared to hope, and believed in the possibility of healing, this workbook is dedicated to you.

May these pages offer connection, strength, and the assurance that you are not alone—and that change is possible.

Table of Contents

Preface

This workbook is a companion to *I Hate Myself*, published in 2025. It is designed to guide you through the challenge of replacing self-hatred with self-compassion. As a therapist, I have seen the exhausting weight of self-hatred. It impacts your relationships, undermines your accomplishments, and tells you that you are fundamentally flawed. You may have lived with these feelings for so long that it feels like an unchangeable part of who you are. *It isn't.* Self-hatred is learned—and that means it can be unlearned.

The process isn't easy, but you can reclaim your life from self-hatred. I've designed this workbook to serve two complementary purposes. First, it functions as a practical extension of the concepts explored in *I Hate Myself*, which discusses strategies and approaches for overcoming self-hatred, while helping you understand the theory behind the practice. Second, and perhaps most importantly, it provides a framework for therapeutic work—a shared roadmap that you and your therapist can navigate together.

This workbook follows the structure of *I Hate Myself*, so each chapter here corresponds to the same-numbered chapter there. The material in this workbook summarizes the key concepts and builds on them, offering new activities for you to practice these therapeutic techniques. These activities are designed to be revisited and gradually integrated into how you think and feel about yourself. You will notice that some activities overlap or encourage you to retread similar exercises. This repetition is by design. Overcoming self-hatred involves altering your ingrained patterns of thinking, which takes time and practice. Eventually, you will learn new behaviors, skills, and thoughts, which can replace the harmful ones that self-loathing creates and perpetuates. Some activities will resonate immediately; others may feel uncomfortable, unhelpful, or even triggering. This variability is normal and expected. I encourage you to work through this material at a pace that feels manageable, always in consultation with your therapist, who can help you process what arises.

Self-hatred often accompanies conditions like depression, anxiety, borderline personality disorder, and eating disorders. If you're managing any of these conditions, know that addressing self-hatred is not separate from your treatment—it's a part of it. By developing self-compassion and understanding, many people find that they can change their thoughts and behaviors in a positive way.

Throughout this workbook, you'll be asked to examine your core beliefs, let go of self-blame, and make space to give your future self a better and more compassionate life. I hope this workbook helps you take those vital, and sometimes daunting, first steps toward realizing that you have been wrong about who you are and in so doing replace all the negative lessons of your past with a deep and enduring kindness toward yourself.

Please note that there are some suggestions for the therapist scattered throughout the book. I've set these in italics to make them easy to spot.

—Blaise Aguirre

Part 1

Understanding Self-Hatred

The purpose of this workbook is to discuss self-hatred with your therapist so you can work through it together. Before reading Chapters 1–5 in this workbook, review the Part 1 Activity, which will help you frame your thoughts and make a plan to address your feelings in therapy.

Part 1 Activity: Bringing Up Self-Hatred in Therapy

You cannot work on self-hatred if you don't bring it up in therapy. Even if you are not in therapy, recognize that it is a problem that is not fixed in you and be willing to address it. Reflect on the following questions to prepare for your next conversation with your therapist.

- Have you ever discussed self-hatred with your therapist?

____

____

____

____

- If not, what has made it difficult to do so?

____

____

____

____

- What is your concern about what will happen if you bring it up?

- Are you convinced that it is something that will never change?

- Can you make a commitment to yourself to bring it up at least once in your next therapy session?

- Write down your next therapy appointment date and time, and your commitment to bring up your self-hatred then. If saying the words out loud is too uncomfortable, show your commitment note to your therapist to help you get started.

Chapter 1

What Is Self-Hatred?

Chapter Summary

Self-hatred is a persistent and intense dislike of the self. It comes with feelings of inadequacy, shame, guilt, self-blame, and low self-worth. This is not a state of mind that will improve on its own, and it's far more than what a person feels when they mess up or react to an accident they've made. When a person with self-loathing makes a mistake, they perceive it as proof that they are inadequate and undeserving. Their embarrassment and self-criticism will stick with them as they struggle to move past the event.

Self-hatred, and the thought and emotional patterns it generates, become a deep and painful problem that impacts all aspects of life. It evolves to become embedded in an individual's core sense of self directing their inner dialogue. It is related to self-criticism, self-disgust, self-blame, and self-contempt, but self-hatred is distinct and doesn't always overlap with these constructs.

Key Definitions and Concepts

- **Self-hatred:** A persistent core belief of being unworthy, bad, or broken.
- **Self-criticism:** The tendency to engage in negative self-evaluation that results in feelings of worthlessness; historically linked to depression.
- **Self-disgust:** A sense of disgust or revulsion directed toward the self, either physically or behaviorally.
- **Self-blame:** The act of attributing the consequences of an experience to a person's own actions or character; also connected to an inflated sense of control.

- **Self-contempt:** A clinical phenomenon that interferes with emotional processing and leads to a person's active rejection or scorn for some aspect of the self that seems alien or not a part of them.
- **Trauma response:** An emotional response to a harmful or life-threatening event like an accident, crime, natural disaster, abuse, or violence. Trauma can have a lasting negative impact on a person's function and well-being.
- **Core beliefs:** A person's individual perspective that influences how they see the world and themselves.

Despite it feeling so for those with lived experience, self-hatred is not an innate part of human beings. It is an erroneous and yet painfully enduring sense of self that can develop over time, in response to deep feelings of inadequacy and shame, created by enduring messaging that teach the person that they are inadequate and deserving of little, including love. The most important thing to understand about self-hatred is that it is *not* a natural part of any human. It is a toxic false narrative that feels true and certain to the person experiencing it. We know this in part because self-loathing does not typically respond to standard approaches such as cognitive behavioral therapy (CBT), dialectical behavior therapy (DBT), or others, and nor does it respond to medications. It is a learned and ingrained concept and behavior rather than a biological condition, although it may be linked to mental health conditions.

Chapter 1 Warmup Activity: Differentiating Related Concepts

The first step to overcoming your self-hatred is to better understand it. Complete the following table to determine how and how often self-hatred and related concepts affect your life.

Concept	Definition	Personal Example	Frequency (Rarely/ Occasionally/Frequently)
Self-hatred	A persistent core belief of being unworthy, bad, or broken		
Self-criticism	Negative self-evaluation about specific actions or traits		
Self-disgust	Revulsion toward one's body or behaviors		
Self-blame	Attributing problems to one's own actions or character		
Self-contempt	Active scorn or rejection of aspects of self		

1. Which of these do you experience most often?

____

____

____

____

2. Which feels most painful or persistent?

____

____

____

____

Core Versus Transient Self-Hatred

There are two main ways self-hatred presents. Core self-hatred describes a person's enduring experience, while transient self-hatred is an emotional response. Core self-hatred has five features:

1. **Deeply ingrained:** Typically develops and ingrains in early childhood in the context of deeply hurtful and invalidating experiences.
2. **Identity level:** Feels like a fundamental truth about the self.
3. **Persistent:** Does not easily fade or respond to positive feedback or positive accomplishments.
4. **Linked to mental health conditions:** These include chronic depression, complex post-traumatic stress disorder (PTSD), and borderline personality disorder.
5. **Self-perpetuating:** Behaviors tend to be consistent with the belief, for example, avoiding growth opportunities and repeatedly engaging in toxic relationships—behaviors that reinforce the belief.

Not commonly a presenting symptom: Because the person has always felt this way, it is the only way that they know their life. If a person has always had a headache, that is their enduring experience, and so they do not know that it is a problem. However, when someone has not had a headache in one moment, they then notice a headache when it appears.

I Hate Myself was primarily focused on core self-hatred. This affects a person's life by making them believe they are a significant burden to those around them. These thoughts are often tied to early trauma and invalidation during childhood. The higher the level of core self-hatred, the higher the risk of suicide and suicidal thoughts. Core self-hatred is deeply ingrained and feels like a fundamental truth about someone. It doesn't easily fade, and it is something a person always remembers feeling. It is always self-perpetuating, meaning that a person's behaviors align with their belief that they are a burden. This makes them likely to avoid growth opportunities and engage in toxic relationships. These behaviors, in turn, reinforce the belief that a person is unworthy of love and support. Core self-hatred is linked to mental health conditions such as chronic depression, complex PTSD, and borderline personality disorder.

While core self-hatred presents as a structural part of a person's identity, transient self-hatred tends to present as a reactive cognitive and emotional response.

Transient self-hatred appears intermittently and is often triggered by specific events that are typically outside of a person's control; these feelings come and go based on mood, stress levels, and external conditions. It may be rooted in recent struggles and failures rather than deep, painful childhood experiences. The six features of transient self-hatred are:

1. **Situational:** Tends to be triggered by specific, and typically external events.
2. **Fluctuating:** Comes and goes based on mood, stress, and external conditions.
3. **Not identity level:** Although self-hatred appears to be on a continuum, people with transient self-hatred don't feel self-hatred at their core.
4. **Tends to respond to logic and CBT interventions:** Self-compassion, problem-solving, and mindfulness are more readily accepted.
5. **More common in mental health dips:** Tends not to be as present when the person is doing well and is more present during depression or stress episodes.
6. **More likely to be a presenting complaint:** In contrast to core self-hatred, there is more of a recognition that it is a problem that needs to be addressed.

Transient self-hatred commonly appears during mental health dips, fading when the person is doing well. This makes people with transient self-hatred more likely to recognize that it is a problem they should address. While they may have the desire to die during moments of intense self-hatred, suicidal desires or thoughts aren't as persistent or intense as those tied to core self-hatred. Despite this, they are distressing. Transient self-hatred is more likely to

Table 1.1 Core Versus Transient Self-Hatred

	Core	Transient
Duration and consistency	It's always there no matter what.	It comes in waves: sometimes there sometimes not.
Trigger/prompt dependency	It's always there even on "good days."	It spikes after specific events.
Belief flexibility	You don't believe people who tell you that you are loveable.	You recognize that you might have been treating yourself too harshly.
Impact on behavior	You avoid opportunities and enter into predictably toxic relationships.	You might withdraw temporarily but tend to bounce back.
Childhood trauma/history	It's often tied to early trauma and invalidation.	It may be rooted in recent struggles and failures.

respond to logic and CBT interventions. People with transient self-hatred are more likely to accept self-compassion, problem-solving, and mindfulness as ways to manage thoughts of self-loathing.

Table 1.1 summarizes the differences between core and transient self-hatred.

The Development of a Sense of Self

The question of how self-hatred develops and evolves is an important theme in considering its development, and a quick overview of child development is helpful.

The development of a child's individual sense of self is a complex and continuous process that begins at birth and is heavily influenced by their interactions with the world and the people around them. It involves recognizing themselves as distinct from others, recognizing their own thoughts and feelings, on their way to developing a unique identity.

From infancy to early childhood, and depending on a child's temperament and level of attunement[1] and awareness, their self-concept starts with how adults

[1]Attunement is the ability to sense and respond accurately to another person's emotional state, creating a feeling of being understood, validated, and safe.

respond to them. Fundamental connection through warm, caring interactions, good eye contact, and listening with curiosity leads to the creation of a healthy emotional bond, which is crucial for a healthy self-concept. When caregivers consistently and predictably meet an infant's needs, the child develops a sense of trust and security, which is foundational to feeling safe enough to explore their own identity. Around 18 months, toddlers begin to recognize themselves in mirrors and photographs. This "mirror self-recognition" is a significant milestone, indicating the emergence of a reflective self and laying the groundwork for self-conscious emotions like embarrassment and pride.

As language develops, toddlers start using "me" and "my," asserting their individuality and growing sense of autonomy. They begin to identify with their name as a unique label. As the child gets older, adults sharing memories and stories about the child's past helps them construct an internal picture of themselves over time, forming their "autobiography." As the child develops and becomes increasingly self-aware, they learn to identify and name their own emotions and understand how their feelings influence their behavior. This is crucial for emotional regulation and empathy.

If a child continues in a healthy, empathic and validating environment, even a highly sensitive child should continue to develop in emotionally healthy ways, but it is during these early years that the seeds of self-hatred can be planted. A child's individual sense of self is not something they are born with. And certainly, any sense of sense of self that might exist is not at all fully formed. Their sense of self is continuously constructed and refined through a dynamic interplay of their innate biology, their experiences, and their relationships with the world around them.

Children are *not* born hating themselves. It is something they learn. It is critical to understand this idea in order to overcome self-hatred. Once a person realizes that they were not born hating themselves, but that they learned to do so, then they realize that they can learn to love themselves.

The Role of Core Beliefs

If self-hatred isn't a natural part of some unlucky human beings and isn't depression, then where does it come from? There is evidence that self-loathing has its roots in a person's culture, childhood experiences, and familial interactions. It can also arise from trauma. Any significant experience—such as early childhood experiences, family interactions, social and cultural influences, and trauma—can form or shape a person's core beliefs.

Many of our core beliefs are established in childhood, when we are learning about the world and considering our role in it. Over time, these beliefs shape our sense of self and how we interpret our relationships.

The following activities are designed for anyone to complete with their therapist. If you are working independently, you should be able to use all of these activities on your own; however, a therapist would be able to recommend specific techniques and strategies to help you more effectively address your feelings. CBT and DBT work best when you practice them with the guidance of a trained therapist.

Activity 1.1: Self-Hatred Questionnaire

Self-hatred has varying degrees. To better understand how you experience it, answer the following questions. For each question, score your response using a 1–5 scale, where:

1 = Strongly disagree

2 = Disagree

3 = Neutral

4 = Agree

5 = Strongly agree

Questions

1. I feel intense dislike for myself. *Score:* _____
2. I am disgusted with myself. *Score:* _____
3. I feel like I am a bad person. *Score:* _____
4. I do not deserve kindness or compassion. *Score:* _____
5. I get angry at myself for things I do or think. *Score:* _____
6. I wish I could change who I am. *Score:* _____
7. I feel like I am a failure. *Score:* _____

To find your total score, add your responses for all seven items.

Total score: _____

The lowest possible score is 7. The highest possible score is 35. Higher scores indicate greater self-hatred. People with transient self-hatred might be able to guess that their score would be different if they completed the questionnaire on a different day because their mood and circumstances heavily influence their level of self-loathing. People with core self-hatred will feel confident that their scores will be the same, regardless of when they answer the questions.

Activity 1.2: Your Core Beliefs

Complete the table to better understand the core beliefs that determine how you perceive the world. Then, answer the questions to reflect on how your core beliefs impact your life and your sense of self-hatred.

My Perspective	**What I Think Others See**
Describe the kind of person you are. *I am . . .*	Describe how you think other people would describe you. *Other people think I am . . .*
Think about what you like most about yourself. *I love myself when . . .*	Consider what you believe other people like most about you. *People love me when I . . .*

Consider what you bring into the world and what your purpose is.

My role in the world is . . .

Consider your thoughts about other people believe about your purpose in the world.

People see my purpose is . . .

Reflect on how you see the world and other people. Include your reasoning.

The world . . .

Reflect: The purpose of our core belief system is to provide us the underlying structure for interpreting reality, regulating our emotions, and guiding actions, and this profoundly impacts our overall mental health, relationships, and life satisfaction. If core beliefs are limiting instead of supportive, it is time to change them.

1. Based on your answers, what are your core beliefs about yourself?

2. What are your core beliefs about the world?

3. How do you think those core beliefs contribute to your self-hatred?

____

____

____

____

4. How do those core beliefs impact your relationships?

____

____

____

____

5. Which core beliefs have a negative impact on your life?

____

____

____

____

6. What would it take for you to change those core beliefs?

____

____

____

____

Activity 1.3: Echoes of the Past

We all carry our past experiences with us and they shape who we are and how we think about ourselves and the world. Now that you better understand your current core beliefs, take a moment to determine where they came from. With your therapist, answer the following questions to connect your core beliefs to your past experiences. This will help you understand how experience can feed your self-hatred.

Reflection: These questions help you identify and acknowledge early messages you believed about yourself.

1. What messages did you receive about yourself from caregivers, teachers, or peers when you were young?

___

___

___

___

2. Write down your experiences of feeling criticized or belittled.

___

___

___

___

3. Who were the people who criticized or belittled you?

___

___

___

___

4. How do you think those messages have shaped your core beliefs about yourself?

___

___

___

___

5. Have you experienced past trauma that has impacted your core beliefs? If so, what happened, and what did you learn about yourself and the world? How has that trauma influenced your core beliefs?

___

___

___

___

Exploration: These questions challenge you to think about different types of messages you may have overlooked.

6. How old were you when you first had the experience of self-hatred?

____

____

____

____

7. Do you recall a time when you felt loved and important?

____

____

____

____

8. Did you think of yourself as different from other children? If so, how?

____

____

____

____

Your core beliefs are echoes of the past that feed your self-loathing, but they are not a part of *you*. You are not the same person you were when these things happened to you, and you are more than the sum of what you have experienced. Once you accept that you have the innate power to change your core beliefs, you will be one step closer to changing them.

Activity 1.4: Challenging the Narrative

Cognitive restructuring is a core component of CBT, and therapists use it to address various mental health conditions. It is a therapeutic technique used to identify and change negative or irrational thought patterns to improve mental well-being. It works by challenging and modifying these thoughts, often by replacing them with more balanced or positive ones. Answer the following questions to regain a more realistic and balanced perspective.

1. Assume that self-hatred is a lie that was taught to you. What evidence do you have that supports your self-hatred belief? What evidence do you have that invalidates it?

____

____

____

____

2. Recognizing that we all have flaws, what is a more balanced way to see yourself? Write down a few neutral or even positive parts of who you are.

____

____

____

____

3. What would you say to a friend who had your experiences and beliefs about self-hatred?

____

____

____

____

4. Describe a situation that elicited strong self-hatred. Imagine that you discuss this situation with a caring friend or compassionate therapist and take on their point of view. What do they say to you to help you stop judging yourself so harshly?

____

____

____

____

To practice these techniques, work with your therapist to have a dialogue using role-play:

1. Review a situation that elicited strong self-hatred. For instance, say you are late for therapy, and you are judging yourself.

____

____

____

____

2. Your therapist expresses compassion and alternative perspectives.

____

____

____

____

3. Now, you role-play a friend who is late, and the therapist pretends to be you.

____

____

____

____

This can help you become more accustomed to hearing and considering these new perspectives, making you more flexible in your own thinking.

Activity 1.5: Guided Journaling

Journaling can have many therapeutic benefits. Writing about your experiences can help you regulate and process emotions and trauma by helping you work through complex feelings. Writing down your feelings can also reduce their intensity and bring clarity to your experiences by creating psychological distance. This can make them seem more manageable by interrupting negative thought patterns and rumination. Rumination is when a person gets stuck in a mental loop that leads them to over-analyze situations and obsess over perceived mistakes or failures. These repetitive thoughts can amplify negative emotions because they focus on problems instead of solutions. This can make it harder to find solutions or move past painful events.

Take your time to write responses to the following prompts. Taking a different perspective will help you focus on things that encourage self-compassion.

1. List three traits or characteristics that are totally separate from your self-hatred (e.g., "I am curious," "I am resilient," "I am a good friend.").

   ____

   ____

   ____

   ____

2. Recall a time when you showed strength or kindness, even if it felt small.

   ____

   ____

   ____

   ____

Activity 1.6: Overly Self-Critical Thinking

Overly self-critical thinking perpetuates self-hatred by creating a vicious cycle where negative thoughts reinforce painful emotions, which then fuel even harsher self-judgment. This is because every self-attack, for example, "I'm so stupid," triggers shame, which perpetuates the person's feeling of being inherently flawed. Then, harsh and negative self-talk frames mistakes as moral failures "because I am stupid," instead of as fixable problems, which would sound like, "I was exhausted and didn't fully understand, and I can always ask others for help." Finally, because the person is harshly judging themselves, they tend to believe that others judge them, too, and any failure is seen as deserving punishment from the self and others.

Describe a recent mistake and answer the following questions:

1. How did you talk to yourself about it?

2. What did I say to myself?

3. Was I fair or overly harsh?

4. What emotions showed up?

5. What would I say to a friend in the same situation?

Key Points

- Self-hatred is a learned set of behaviors or feelings that can be unlearned. Change is possible.
- Self-hatred is not an innate part of a person. It comes from many outside factors.
- Our core beliefs influence our perspective on the world and on ourselves. These beliefs are not fixed and permanent. When they no longer serve us, we should revise them to help us have a more positive outlook on ourselves, the future, and the people around us.
- Childhood experiences and family relationships send and reinforce messages that can lead to limiting core beliefs.
- Trauma has lingering effects on our thinking by undermining our self-worth and strengthening core beliefs that limit us. This is our mind's attempt to protect us from more harm, but it often results in self-criticism and negative thinking patterns that reduce trust and damage relationships.
- By changing our core beliefs, we can shift our perspective on the world to see ourselves as valuable and worthy participants. We can all learn self-compassion.

Chapter 2

Why Is Overcoming Self-Hatred So Critical?

Chapter Summary

There are two extremely serious reasons why self-hatred should be addressed. First, the lived experience is debilitating. Second, it is a strong risk factor for suicide. Self-hatred is emotionally painful, limiting, and pervasive. It can significantly and negatively impact relationships, making it difficult to form and maintain healthy connections. It can destroy a person's confidence, impacting their ability to perform at work or school. People with self-loathing can struggle with intimacy, trust, and communication, often believing that they are unlovable or a burden to others. This can lead to a cycle of negativity, insecurity, and enduring relationship conflict.

Key Definitions and Concepts

- **Suicidal ideation:** Thoughts, considerations, and a preoccupation with the idea of death and suicide. These thoughts may come and go, or be extremely distracting. Some people go so far as planning a way to take their lives.
- **Self-harm:** When a person intentionally hurts their own body on purpose. Self-harm doesn't typically present with suicidal ideation.
- **Inner critic:** The thoughts and judgments that emerge from self-criticism.
- **Lived experience:** An individual's subjective, personal reality. The lived experience occurs as a person directly experiences the world and makes sense of it.

I repeat, suicide is *not* a solution to self-hatred. Neither is self-harm nor living with this chronic symptom. Working together, we can help everyone to directly address their self-hatred and see the potential they possess.

Chapter 2 Warmup Activity: Your Lived Experience

Read this excerpt from someone living with self-hatred, then answer the following questions:

> *It's really hard to even think of a friendship or relationship where I have felt totally secure because of constantly hating myself for everything I think is wrong about me... Every single time I've ever had a job interview or taken a test or interacted with a friend, I leave those situations with the voice in my brain telling me that I suck, and I hate myself in one way or another.*

1. Can you relate to any part of this experience? Which parts and how so?

____

____

____

____

2. If you had to describe your self-hatred in a few sentences, what would you write?

____

____

____

____

If you don't want self-hatred to have such a negative impact on your life, you have to address it. Keep these reflections in mind when as you read the rest of this chapter and answer the questions at the end.

Self-Hatred and Suicidal Thoughts

Research shows that self-hatred is a strong predictor of suicidal ideation. Some studies reveal that people with self-hatred are suicidal because they believe that they are a burden to others, and/or because they feel alone, and that they don't to any group. Other studies suggest that suicidal thoughts function as a way to escape painful or unwanted emotions. Suicide is *not* a solution.

Some people with self-hatred also engage in self-harm, deliberately injuring themselves. Research shows that people who self-harm and also have a psychiatric diagnosis are more likely to report more emotional abuse and more self-hatred. Childhood abuse had a particularly strong emotional impact, and self-hatred worsened this.

Self-hatred can also impact various aspects of self-care. For instance, people with eating disorders often struggle with markedly low self-esteem and are at risk for suicidal behavior. they also often experience perceived burdensomeness, which is a vulnerability factor for suicidal behaviors. Specifically, and as discussed in *I Hate Myself*, when perceived burdensomeness, which is comprised of self-hate and the sense of being a liability to others, is present, suicidal thoughts and behaviors must be evaluated.

If you have thoughts of suicide or self-harm, contact a therapist or counselor immediately and get help from someone who cares about you. Here are a few resources to help you get help fast:

- Suicide and Crisis Lifeline: Text or call 988 or chat at 988lifeline.org.
- Emergency Services: Call 911 or your local emergency services if danger or self-harm seem imminent.

Some have asked if self-hatred is simply a form of depression, but these are separate entities, even if they can co-occur. However, they also commonly co-occur. In the context of depression, activities of daily living (ADLs) can become overwhelming, and many people allow their basic needs, including personal hygiene, dressing, and eating, to go unfulfilled. Not addressing these needs can worsen depression and the overall sense of self. This creates a bidirectional relationship where depression affects ADLs in ways that make depression worse. When we fail to take care of ourselves, it can lead to increasing isolation. This can worsen feelings of self-hatred and loneliness.

The Inner Critic

Self-criticism is the tendency to negatively evaluate yourself, and it often results in feelings of worthlessness or depression. It is often automatic and unconscious, but it is highly destructive. The inner critic is the personification of this concept.

When a person engages in self-criticism, they give their inner critic voice, which can result in pervasive negative thoughts and distortions in perception. In addition to depression, it is linked to perfectionism, anxiety, borderline personality disorder, post-traumatic stress disorder, eating disorders, imposter syndrome, and other mental health conditions.

Many high performers have higher levels of self-criticism because they set high standards and can be relentless in their pursuit of perfection. Despite any success they might create, the inner critic can lead to unhealthy patterns of thinking. It can leave people feeling inadequate, regardless of their accomplishments. In extreme cases, when a person doesn't live up to the impossible expectations set by their inner critic, they can feel worthless and depressed.

Despite its potentially negative role, the inner critic has a purpose. It can set high standards for people, which can help them set and pursue important goals. It can also help a person avoid failure or embarrassment by identifying threats in their environment. However, when the inner critic fuels intense self-criticism and self-hatred, it is no longer helpful. Cognitive and dialectical behavioral therapy can help replace or redirect harmful self-criticisms, allowing a person to use positive thinking to reach their goals and free themselves from self-loathing.

Often, you can find evidence in daily life that contradicts your self-criticism. When you begin to look for signs that your inner critic is wrong, you are likely to find them. Looking past the emotional pain of your lived experience can be hard, but it can help you take a more objective viewpoint. This can help you understand that much of your self-criticism is fueled more by pervasive and debilitating thoughts than reality.

Work through the following activities with your therapist. They can give you a starting point for quieting your inner critic and improving your lived experience.

Activity 2.1: Mapping the Effects of Self-Hatred

Reflect on your current life, relationships, routine, and habits, and the role self-hatred plays. Then, complete the following table, giving one or two recent examples from your life to more clearly recognize your lived experience.

	How Self-Hatred Shows Up—Examples	Impact/Consequences
Relationships		
Interactions and relationships with family, friends, and romantic partners		
Work/school		
Choice of job or school		
Tolerance of devaluing behavior from colleagues or classmates		
Ability to persevere during difficult moments such as work evaluations or exams		
Self-care/health		
Personal hygiene		
Eating habits and behaviors		
Impact on relationships and self-esteem		

(continued)

(continued)

Hobbies and enjoyment	
Activities/hobbies you enjoy	
Activities that you don't enjoy but do, simply to make other people happy	

Activity 2.2: The Voice of Self-Hatred

Reflect on what your inner critic sounds like at its worst and write down some of the most common negative thoughts you have about yourself. For each one, note how often it appears and if there are specific emotions that show up with the thoughts.

Self-Hating Thought	Frequency (Rare/Often/Always)	Emotional Impact

Activity 2.3: Challenging the Narrative

You do not need to accept what your inner critic says. To challenge the narrative, replace thoughts that don't serve you well with more positive ones that can help you regain control of your thinking. This isn't easy, but planning, repetition, and reinforcement will help.

For each self-hating thought you wrote in Activity 2.2, write a compassionate alternative response. If you have trouble coming up with things, imagine what you would say to someone you love if they expressed these thoughts. Or, think about positive things people in your life have said or done that proves that the self-hating thought isn't always true.

Example

Self-hating thought: "I am a burden to everyone."

Alternative: "Some people have told me they care about me and value my friendship."

Self-Hating Thought	Alternative

Activity 2.4: Coping When Suicidal Thoughts Are Loud

Many people with lived experience can have suicidal thoughts and behaviors, and this is supported by research that shows that many people with self-hatred feel that they are a burden to others. If self-hatred has led to thoughts of self-harm or suicide, use this space to identify warning signs, triggers, and coping strategies. It is also important to have a list of supportive people or resources to contact in times of crisis.

When self-hatred is very strong and suicidal thoughts become louder, make a list of your:

1. **Warning signs:** *(e.g., social isolation and withdrawal, irritability, etc.)*

   ____

   ____

   ____

   ____

2. **Trigger situations:** *(e.g., certain people, certain interactions, etc.)*

   ____

   ____

   ____

   ____

3. **Coping strategies:** *(e.g., distress tolerance skills from DBT, TIPP as described in the appendix)*

   ____

   ____

   ____

   ____

4. **Supportive contacts:** *Include your individual therapist, supportive parent/family member, friend, colleague, etc.*

   ____

   ____

   ____

   ____

5. **If urges are overwhelming:** *When do you call emergency services? Who is your MUST-go-to person?*

____

____

____

____

When you first recognize the warning signs or trigger situations, follow your plan.

Key Points

- Self-hatred is strongly linked to suicidal ideation, self-harm, and suicide. If you experience thoughts like these, contact a therapist or counselor immediately. Ask for help from people in your life who you care about.
- Self-hatred can have a negative impact on all aspects of life, including relationships, work, and basic self-care.
- Your inner critic is the voice of self-hatred.
- While the inner critic can serve a valuable purpose, especially for high-performers, it if isn't counterbalanced, it can lead to pervasive negative thought patterns.
- Try to counterbalance your inner critic by considering what you actually see, hear, and experience in the moment. Often, these aspects of life prove your inner critic wrong.
- Prepare a plan to help you cope with difficult thoughts.

Chapter 3

Common Signs of Self-Hatred

Chapter Summary

While self-hatred impacts every person's life in a different way, there are common signs that many people with self-loathing share. As mentioned in Chapter 3 of *I Hate Myself*, most therapists do not screen for self-hatred in their initial evaluations. As a result, people with feelings of self-hatred do not typically bring up the topic on their own, so this source of suffering is often overlooked in therapy.

Key Definitions and Concepts

- **Cognitive distortion:** A pattern of thinking that is based on inaccurate or irrational beliefs.
- **All-or-nothing thinking:** A cognitive distortion where someone views people, experiences, or situations in terms of extreme absolutes without considering the full range of possibilities.
- **Emotional reasoning:** Equating emotion with fact, so that you draw conclusions based on how you feel instead of what is actually happening.
- **Chain analysis:** A tool in dialectical behavior therapy (DBT) that can help you understand behavior by tracking a sequence of events: the antecedent, the behavior, and the consequences. Together, these make up the ABC model of chain analysis.

Recognizing the signs of your self-hatred can help you minimize its presence in your life. To begin this chapter, develop a plan to describe your self-hatred to your therapist, if you haven't already done so.

Chapter 3 Warmup Activity: Start the Conversation About Self-Hatred

Answer the following questions to raise the issue of self-hatred with your therapist.

1. Have you discussed self-hatred with your therapist?

2. If so, what terms have you used to describe it? *Self-hatred? Self-loathing?*

3. Do you think your therapist understands what you are experiencing?

4. If not, how can you better explain how self-hatred impacts your life? Write down what you plan to say.

5. If you haven't discussed self-hatred with your therapist, what would make you feel comfortable bringing it up?

____

____

____

____

It is worth addressing your self-hatred so it no longer has such a negative impact on your life. Keep these reflections in mind as you read the rest of this chapter and answer the questions at the end.

Cognitive Distortions

Self-hatred is often driven by negative thinking patterns that become automatic habits that direct how a person feels, how they evaluate their behavior, and what they believe about the attitudes and motives of other people. Some of these thinking patterns are cognitive distortions, which are inaccurate and systematic ways a person interprets the world. We discussed some of these—and related thinking patterns—in Chapter 3 of *I Hate Myself* because they can be signs of self-hatred.

For most of us, thoughts are automatic, repetitive, and mindless. Many people with profound self-hatred struggle with cognitive distortions, and it is an important step in treatment for patients to recognize these as they arise. The teaching point for patients is that cognitive distortions are irrational or exaggerated thought patterns that reinforce negative thinking and emotions. When these distortions become habitual, they can perpetuate self-hatred by creating a vicious cycle of self-criticism, shame, and hopelessness.

You may not consciously realize that cognitive distortions influence your thoughts. For example, imagine you are going to the grocery store and have a long list of things you need to buy. On your way out the door, your spouse asks you to pick up a box of their favorite breakfast cereal. You say you will, then forget as soon as you get in the car. You didn't write the cereal down on your list and don't remember to buy it. When you get home, your spouse asks if you got their cereal. You immediately feel a surge of guilt, shame, and self-loathing. You say, "I'm so sorry. I can't believe I forgot! I screw up everything. I don't even know why you stay married to me. I'm a terrible partner." Even a few days later, you feel overwhelmed by your thoughts and emotions. In this instance, a simple oversight, forgetting to buy cereal, becomes evidence that you are a failure, a terrible spouse, and undeserving of love.

Recognizing the Signs of Self-Hatred

Cognitive distortions are behind many of the signs of self-hatred, but they aren't the only way to notice how self-loathing affects your self-esteem and relationships. The signs of self-hatred can be difficult to notice unless you are looking for them. Here is a recap of the signs from Chapter 3 of *I Hate Myself*:

- **All-or-nothing thinking:** Viewing situations in extreme terms without recognizing any middle ground.
- **Focusing on the negative:** The tendency to see the drawbacks or bad side of every situation.
- **Emotional reasoning:** The experience of having a feeling, then coming to a conclusion about a situation based solely on that feeling.
- **Seeking approval and constant reassurance:** Looking for constant reassurance, which could mean that you cannot find a sense of confidence or validation yourself.
- **Refusal to accept compliments:** This is a sign that you discount your accomplishments, believing that they aren't worthy of praise, or perhaps you believe that the people offering praise are not sincere.
- **Doing all you can to fit in:** Going against your own values or genuine interests to avoid feeling lonely.
- **Taking any sort of feedback as criticism or a personal attack:** When you lack self-confidence, feedback can feel like criticism and eclipse compliments and generate negative feelings long after it is shared.
- **Bringing others down:** Intentionally making other people feel bad and not being able to stand when someone else is happy.
- **Fearing healthy connections:** Pushing others away out of a fear that they will discover what an awful person you are and leave. Sometimes people

who fear healthy connections also accept unacceptable behavior from others because they don't believe they deserve better.

- **Being afraid of having, or refusing to have, big dreams and goals:** The belief that nothing will work out and that you will inevitably fail.
- **Being overly self-critical:** Blaming yourself and refusing to be self-compassionate, even after making small mistakes or failing due to outside circumstances.

After years or decades of living with these thoughts and habitual behaviors, they can become almost invisible, operating on a subconscious level to reinforce your negative beliefs about yourself and others.

Table 3.1 offers examples of how specific cognitive distortions can contribute to self-hatred. Add your experiences to the list of distortions that apply to your lived experience.

Table 3.1 Cognitive Distortions and Self-Hatred

Cognitive Distortion and an Example	How It Fuels Self-Hatred	Effect
All-or-nothing thinking *"If I'm not perfect, I'm worthless."*	Viewing yourself as either a complete success or a total failure.	Small mistakes feel catastrophic, reinforcing self-loathing.
Overgeneralization *"I failed at this, so I fail at everything."*	Taking one negative event as evidence that everything about you is bad.	Creates a sense of hopelessness and worthlessness.

(continued)

Table 3.1 *(continued)*

Cognitive Distortion and an Example	How It Fuels Self-Hatred	Effect
Mental filtering (negative bias) *"I had a great review at work, but the areas I need to improve on prove that I'm a terrible employee."*	Focusing only on flaws while ignoring strengths.	Distorts self-perception, making self-hatred feel justified.
Disqualifying the positive *"They only said I did well to be nice—it doesn't count."*	Dismissing compliments or achievements as irrelevant.	Maintains a negative self-image despite evidence to the contrary.
Jumping to conclusions (mind reading & fortune telling) *"No one responded to my texts because they think I'm pathetic."*	Assuming others hate you or that you'll always fail.	Reinforces feelings of rejection and unworthiness.

Cognitive Distortion and an Example	How It Fuels Self-Hatred	Effect
Magnification (catastrophizing) & minimization *"My mistake ruined everything (but my successes don't matter)."*	Blowing up flaws while downplaying strengths.	Keeps self-worth tied to perceived failures.
Emotional reasoning *"I feel like a failure, so I must be one."*	Believing any thoughts that arise during strong emotions to being factual truths.	Confirms self-hatred based on emotions alone.
"Should" statements *"I should always be productive; otherwise, I'm lazy."*	Punishing yourself for not meeting unrealistic standards.	Leads to guilt, shame, and self-punishment.

(continued)

Table 3.1 *(continued)*

Cognitive Distortion and an Example	How It Fuels Self-Hatred	Effect
Labeling *"I'm stupid and worthless."*	Defining yourself by mistakes with harsh labels.	Solidifies a negative self-identity.
Personalization *"It's all my fault they're upset."*	Blaming yourself for things outside your control.	Increases self-blame and shame.

These common cognitive distortions should be reviewed regularly so that when they arise in therapy and life outside of therapy in the future, the patient becomes expert in labeling the distortions, catching them earlier and thereby preventing them from becoming repetitive ruminations. Beyond distortions, there are also behaviors that reinforce self-hatred, and it is an important step in therapy that patients know all of the thoughts and behaviors that are keeping them stuck.

Fear and Self-Hatred

People who experience self-hatred and have past trauma often fear close connections and big dreams because close connections and hope often trigger memories of the way that closeness was hurtful and how hope was shot down. Table 3.2 summarizes common beliefs driven by fear, and how they impact connections and big dreams. Write down your experiences.

Table 3.2 Fear and Self-Hatred Beliefs

Fear and Self-Hatred Belief	Influence on Connection	Influence on Big Dreams
Rejection and abandonment *"I am unworthy of love, so others will eventually leave me."*	Past hurt and rejection makes the belief of betrayal or rejection feel inevitable.	Dreams require support; you don't trust others (or yourself) enough to believe in them. Dreams require hope, and this is difficult when hope has been eroded by the doubts and dismissal of others. Dreams require aspiration, and it is hard to aspire when you have been led to believe that you won't amount to anything.
Vulnerability *"If they really knew me, they'd hate me."*	Intimacy means exposing your perceived flaws, risking judgment. Shame tells you you're "too broken" to be loved authentically.	Big dreams require self-expression—you fear being seen and failing publicly.

(continued)

Table 3.2 *(continued)*

Fear and Self-Hatred Belief	Influence on Connection	Influence on Big Dreams
Failure *"I don't deserve success, and failing will prove I'm worthless."*	n/a	Cognitive distortions like all-or-nothing thinking make failure feel catastrophic, or discounting the positive leads to the dismissal of any successes. Past experiences may have taught you that effort leads to punishment, not reward.
Disappointing others *"I'll let everyone down, just like I've let myself down."*	There is an automatic assumption that you will hurt others (as you've been hurt) or fail to meet others' expectations.	If you try and fail, you'll confirm your "worthlessness" and "flawedness" to others.
Hope itself *"Hope is dangerous—it only sets me up for pain and failure."*	When you fear hope, you won't even try to develop relationships with others.	Dreams require hope. Without it, there's no way to envision a better life.

Thought distortions can lead to frequent misunderstandings and unnecessary conflict within relationships. These distortions often cause individuals to misinterpret comments, intentions, or behaviors, which can erode trust and openness. For the person with lived experience of self-hatred, many of life's early messages were in fact hurtful, so even helpful feedback can feel negative because it is filtered through the person's cognitive distortions and brings self-loathing to the forefront of the mind. One way of addressing these misunderstandings is the THINK skill from DBT.

Dialectical Behavior Therapy: THINK

In DBT, the THINK skill is used to reduce conflict. When we're feeling emotionally overwhelmed, it can be hard to access the thinking and rational parts of the brain that help us more effectively deal with situations such as feedback and criticism. THINK is the acronym for the skill that can help shift your thoughts away from unhelpful thinking patterns and toward a clearer state of mind. For example, say that your friend believes that everyone hates them. Their evidence is that they received a "mixed review" from their work supervisor. "They say my work isn't good enough," your friend tells you. When you explore further, the supervisor actually said, "Great work, just one tiny edit!" The self-hating brain hears, "I am being judged by my supervisor, and that it is proof of how flawed I am as a person and I likely deserved all the negative things that the reviewer said."

The THINK skill can help a person redirect their thinking so it becomes more grounded in reality. THINK stands for: think, have empathy, interpretations, notice, and kindness. Here is how these elements work together in the example of your friend's supervisor:

- **Think:** Consider the supervisor's role. Think about the purpose of a review. Think about possible benefits they might be getting from the review. As your friend to think about their supervisor withholding the feedback. Would they want to continue to be unaware of something that could be improved?

  ____

  ____

  ____

  ____

- **Have Empathy:** Ask your friend to try to tune into their supervisor's perspective and role. Even try to consider how they are doing. For instance, consider what it must be like to be a supervisor and have to give feedback to a lot of people. Is your friend automatically assuming the worst of the other person? Can they generate empathy for them instead?

  ____

  ____

  ____

  ____

- **Interpretations:** Ask your friend if they tend to assume the worst about their supervisor's intentions. If a person has had a lot of abuse, bullying, criticism, and invalidation, it is understandable that they might be suspicious and mistrustful. Remind them that, in addition to the hurtful people in the world, there are also many who are kind. Unless we know otherwise, giving them the benefit of the doubt is, in most cases, a more effective approach.

  This step has two important considerations:

  - Take your time time to get to know the person without making automatic judgments. If the other person regularly acts in kind and fair ways, it is likely that they will be kind and fair to you, too.
  - If the other person has a reputation for being harsh, negative, and judgmental, then it makes sense that you would be skeptical of their intentions.

  The important point is to NOT judge everyone's intentions as negative. For every negative interpretation, it's a good idea to try to think of at least one positive or benign interpretation of the other person's actions.

- **Notice:** Notice the other person with an open attitude during your interactions. Remember that our minds are prone to filtering out the positive and focusing on the negative. Review the list of distortions and notice when you are falling into a cognitive trap. For instance, your friend should notice when their supervisor is being pleasant. Notice the positive feedback without discounting it. Notice seeing the supervisor as all bad or all good.

____

____

____

____

- **Kindness:** Considering the above, be mindful and try to respond with as much kindness as possible. This doesn't mean excusing bad behaviour, but rather than becoming defensive, use respectful, non-aggressive language. Kindness generally begets kindness. You have experienced unkindness in your life. Being unkind to others is the opposite of how you want to live your life.

____

____

____

____

Understanding the signs of self-hatred can help you address and manage your inner voice and break harmful patterns of thinking. To learn more about the signs of your self-hatred, complete Activity 3.1, then select the activities that explore the behaviors you engage in that reinforce your self-hatred.

Activity 3.1: Knowing the Behaviors That Reinforce Your Self-Hatred

Now that you have reviewed and reflected on these patterns and behaviors, reflect on them one more time. Try to expand on your previous reflections. Review the list of common self-hatred patterns below. For each, write down recent situations where you noticed these patterns in your own thoughts or behaviors.

Pattern/Sign	Recent Example in My Life
All-or-nothing thinking	
Focusing on the negative	
Emotional reasoning	
Seeking approval/reassurance	
Rejecting compliments	
Doing all you can to fit in	
Taking feedback as criticism	
Bringing others down	

Fearing healthy connections

Avoiding big dreams/goals

Being overly self-critical

The next activities drill down on some of these thought patterns and begin to explore alternatives to the thoughts and actions that keep self-hatred central to the person's identity.

Activity 3.2: All-or-Nothing Thinking

Think of a recent situation where you saw things in extremes (e.g., total failure or total success) and answer the following questions:

1. Describe the situation:

2. What was your all-or-nothing thought?

3. Is there a middle ground you didn't see at the time?

4. What would be a more balanced perspective?

Activity 3.3: Focusing on the Negative

Recall a recent event where you focused only on what went wrong. List both the negatives and, with help if needed, any positives.

Event Description	Negatives I Focused On	Positives I Might Have Missed

Activity 3.4: Emotional Reasoning

Describe a time when you let your feelings define the facts of a situation, and answer the following questions:

1. What happened?

2. What emotion did you feel?

3. What conclusion did you draw based only on that feeling?

4. What evidence is there for and against that conclusion?

5. Are there alternative conclusions that are more balanced, more consistent with the facts, and more useful to your overall sense of self?

Activity 3.5: Approval and Compliments

Reassurance isn't inherently bad, but it can become a crutch that keeps the cycle of self-hatred spinning. This is because, for people who are dependent on it, it is not always available. Further, it is not a permanent solution. If it were, the other person would only have to reassure once that they care. For many who are desperate for reassurance, once is not enough, and then they become dependent on it and seek it from others, rather work on forming their own internal sense of value. Of course, it is hard to access self-reassurance when self-hatred dominates.

Another "problem" with the need for reassurance is that many people simply don't believe it! People with self-hatred often say things about others like "They are just being nice," "They don't want to say what they really feel because they don't want to hurt my feelings," or "My parents have to say nice things because they are my parents." Even therapists can be accused of being nice to their clients "because you are being paid," or "only doing it for the money." Targeting reassurance-seeking is important in helping people to overcome self-hatred.

If you notice that you seek constant approval and reassurance from others, answer the following questions:

1. When do you find yourself asking others for reassurance?

____

____

____

____

2. If they reassure you, for how long does their reassurance help?

____

____

____

____

3. What happens when you don't get the reassurance you want?

____

____

____

____

4. What are the downsides to seeking reassurance?

____

____

____

____

5. Rather than relying on reassurance, what could you say to yourself instead?

____

____

____

____

If you notice that you reject compliments, answer the following questions:

1. Write down the last three compliments you received.

____

____

____

____

2. How did you react?

____

____

____

____

3. Did you feel that they were lies? Something that someone had to say? A reflection of the other person not knowing the "real" you?

____

____

____

____

4. What would it be like to accept them as true, even for a moment?

____

____

____

____

Activity 3.6: Masking to Fit In Versus Authenticity

Being flexible when dealing with others is an adaptive skill that allows a person to act differently in different settings. Wearing a bathing suit with friends at the beach and throwing a frisbee makes sense, but doing so in school or a place of worship would not be appropriate behavior. Knowing how and when to behave is important, but it doesn't mean you should mask who you are simply to fit in. For instance, if a person goes to the beach and throws a frisbee, despite hating those activities, just because they want to be a part of a group, they won't necessarily be happy. And they would leave others with the idea that they enjoy throwing a frisbee at the beach.

Masking, or hiding the true self to fit in or avoid rejection, might feel like survival, but over time, it erodes self-worth and fuels self-hatred, and this can be for many reasons such as reinforcing the belief that "my real self is unacceptable." Although going to the beach once could be a great way to connect, continuing to do so, especially if masking is at play, could lead to emotional exhaustion, feeling alienated, and ultimately becoming resentful over time. Masking may prevent genuine connection because there isn't really a shared interest, and this can lead to loneliness. Continuing to mask reinforces masking and makes it more difficult to break the habitual behavior of doing so.

Describe a time you did something just to fit in, even if it went against your preferences or values. Keeping that in mind, answer the following questions:

1. What did you do?

____

____

____

____

2. Why did you do it?

____

____

____

____

3. How did it feel in the moment?

____

____

____

____

4. How did you feel afterward?

____

____

____

____

5. What might you do differently next time?

____

____

____

____

Activity 3.7: Taking Feedback as Criticism

People with self-hatred often interpret neutral or even positive feedback as criticism because their brain is wired to confirm their deepest, most painful belief: "I am not good enough." This distortion happens through several psychological mechanisms such as confirmation bias, which is the brain's way of focusing on anything that aligns with a core belief. Another possible mechanism is because of hypervigilance to threat—considering that any kind of feedback is a set up for an attack. Then, there is all-or-nothing thinking when if the feedback isn't 100% positive, then it is not positive at all.

Think of a recent time when you received feedback and took it as a personal attack. With that situation in mind, answer the following questions:

1. What was the feedback?

 ____

 ____

 ____

 ____

2. How did I interpret it?

 ____

 ____

 ____

 ____

3. Can I think of an alternative explanation for the intention behind the feedback?

 ____

 ____

 ____

 ____

4. How might I respond differently next time?

Activity 3.8: Bringing Others Down

Hating others will never help you stop hating yourself. You can never truly rise to where you want to be by dragging others down to your level of suffering. This exercise is particularly important if you tend to find yourself in these situations regularly.

In this activity, you'll reflect on a time that you brought someone else down due to anger, envy, jealousy, or generally feeling bad about yourself. Answer the following questions to learn more:

1. What was the situation, and who else was involved?

2. What did they say or do that made you feel worse about yourself?

3. In turn, what did you say or do to undermine them, or to try to make them hurt the way you did?

4. How did you feel before and after my actions?

____

____

____

____

5. Is there a more effective way to act when this type of situation happens again?

____

____

____

____

Activity 3.9: Fear of Connection and Big Dreams

Review how past experiences may have impacted your belief that closeness and aspirational goals are possible, then answer the following questions.

Fearing Healthy Connections

1. Is there someone I've pushed away out of fear they'd discover the "real me"?

____

____

____

____

2. What would it be like to let them get closer?

____

____

____

____

Avoiding Big Dreams and Goals

3. What is a dream or goal I've avoided because I didn't believe I deserved it?

4. What small step could I take toward it?

Activity 3.10: Chain Analysis: ABC Model

A chain analysis is a core DBT tool used to understand the sequence of events leading to a problematic behavior. It helps identify triggers, vulnerabilities, and consequences, allowing individuals to develop more effective coping strategies. Apply the ABC model to a behavior linked to your self-hatred.

	Your Example of Self-Hatred Behavior
Antecedents	What were my vulnerabilities? Was I hungry, tired, irritable, or sick? Where was I? Who was there? What thoughts did I have? What emotions? What happened just before the behavior? Link all of these on a time continuum from moment to moment.

(continued)

(continued)

Behavior	What did I do? Fully describe all the self-hating behaviors that showed up, such as critical thoughts and statements, self-punishing behaviors, and so on.
Consequences	What happened after? How did I feel/act? What emotions did I have? What was the impact on my relationships?

1. What early warning signs can I notice next time?

2. What could I do differently at each stage?

Work with your therapist to use your chain analysis to increase your awareness of self-hatred patterns, challenge distorted thinking, and develop more self-compassionate responses. Use the ABC model regularly to break cycles of self-hatred and problematic behaviors.

Key Points

- Cognitive distortions drive many of the behaviors of self-hatred.
- Recognizing the signs of your self-hatred is important because it allows you to redirect your thoughts and change your assumptions.
- In DBT, chain analysis helps you connect the antecedents, behavior, and consequences of problematic behavior. This is the ABC model.
- Fear can prevent you from developing meaningful connections with others and pursuing goals. Common fears among people with self-hatred are the fears of: rejection and abandonment, vulnerability, failure, disappointing others, and hope itself.
- The THINK skill can help you reduce conflict. The letters in THINK stand for: thinking, having empathy, interpreting, noticing, and kindness.

Chapter 4

The Lived Experience: Breaking the Cycle of Self-Hatred

Chapter Summary

Chapter 4 of *I Hate Myself* is titled "The Lived Experience." This workbook chapter focuses on breaking the cycle of self-hatred and improving a person's lived experience. A person's thoughts about themselves directly impact their emotions, and emotions direct their behavior. When a person experiences self-loathing, their thoughts lead to emotions that reflect this view, which in turn direct them to behave in ways that reinforce their negative beliefs about themselves. This can lead to feelings of hopelessness and despair.

A large part of a person's lived experience comes from interacting with others. Self-hatred has a negative impact on relationships because people whose lived experience is driven by self-loathing do not trust that others actually like them or see them for who they are. It can also lead people to tolerate abusive or negative relationships because they do not believe they deserve love and affection.

Key Definitions and Concepts

- **Cycle of self-hatred:** Thoughts lead to emotions, which lead to behaviors, which shape a person's lived experience and their thoughts. This creates a feedback loop that reinforces self-loathing, making it difficult to break the pattern.
- **Lived experience:** What it feels like moment by moment to experience self-hatred and pervasive, intense negative feelings about oneself, which can be hard to describe to others.
- **Psychological flexibility:** A person's ability to adapt thinking and behavior in response to changes in circumstances, goals, and values. This prevents

people from being rigidly locked in by their immediate thoughts and emotions and past experiences.

- **Psychological inflexibility:** This occurs when a person is controlled by their internal experiences, either in the immediate moment or in the past, because they seem to offer some kind of safety or comfort. This makes it difficult to adapt to new circumstances or break negative thought patterns.
- **Resilience:** The ability to adapt, recover, and heal from adversity, trauma, or stress. Rather than avoiding challenges, resilient people are able to experience them and reflect in a way that maintains psychological well-being.
- **Sense of self:** A person's awareness and understanding of their own identity, characteristics, and role in their own experiences and relationships.

Describing the lived experience of self-hatred can help a person experiencing it view it from a different perspective. This can help them to consider that their thoughts and feelings are incorrect, which can lead to emotions that reinforce positive behavior changes and patterns of thinking.

Chapter 4 Warmup Activity: "I Hate Myself"—Examining the Thought

The thought "I hate myself" is just that—a thought, not a fact. How would you define the experience of self-hatred if you had to break down the thought in a descriptive way, including all its elements. How would you explain what you are experiencing to others? Use this worksheet to break down and describe this thought in detail by answering the following questions:

1. What does "I hate myself" mean to you? This is an open-ended question. Over the course of this workbook, you and your therapist should revisit this question over and over.

____

____

____

____

2. When do you notice this thought most often? Are there certain people, certain places, certain interactions, certain emotions, and so on when it shows up more than at other times?

____

____

____

____

3. What are the specific words, images, or memories that come up when self-hatred thoughts show up?

____

____

____

____

4. How would you explain this thought to somebody who has never experienced it.

____

____

____

____

The Cycle of Self-Hatred

According to the National Science Foundation the average person has about 60,000 thoughts per day. A significant portion of these thoughts, around 80 percent, are considered negative, and a large majority, roughly 95 percent, are repetitive, meaning thoughts you are having today tend to be similar to thoughts you had yesterday. The thought "I hate myself" is one of the common repetitive and negative thoughts that people with lived experience have. Not only is it a negative thought, but it is so repetitive that it feels real. When a person states, "I hate myself," they are continuing to encode the thought. It's a vicious cycle.

Thoughts, emotions, and behaviors are deeply connected. They form a feedback loop that shapes our experiences, reactions, and overall mental and physical well-being. Here's how they relate:

- **Thoughts influence emotions:** The way you interpret or think about a situation can spark emotions. For example, interpreting not being asked on a date as a rejection can lead to sadness, while seeing it as an opportunity to go on a different date might foster excitement.
- **Emotions drive behaviors:** Strong emotions can dictate how you act, and these actions are often automatic. In the above example, sadness might lead to withdrawal. Excitement might lead to a new haircut. These actions are usually direct responses to how you feel in the moment.
- **Behaviors reinforce thoughts and emotions:** The way you behave can validate or shift your thoughts and emotions. For example, withdrawing after feeling sad can reinforce the belief that social situations are frightening and not worth it, perpetuating the cycle.

One way to think about these interactions is through the CBT Triangle (Figure 4.1). CBT uses the "cognitive triangle" to visually explain this interconnection:

Unhelpful or negative thoughts often trigger distressing feelings, which can lead to self-defeating behaviors. These behaviors may then reinforce the negative thoughts, creating a loop that's hard to break.

Beyond CBT and DBT, there are important ideas from other therapies including acceptance and commitment therapy (ACT). ACT can help undo

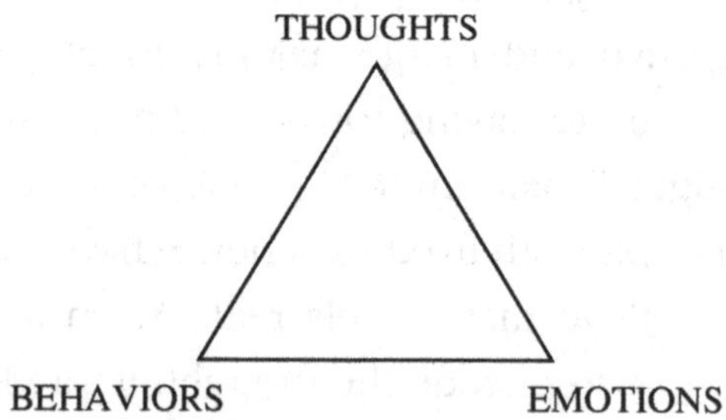

Figure 4.1 Thoughts ↔ Emotions ↔ Behaviors. Each element influences the others in powerful ways.

repeated patterns and is designed to help people manage difficult thoughts and feelings—including negative narratives like self-hatred—by helping them develop psychological flexibility. This means that rather than trying to eliminate or change negative thoughts directly, ACT focuses on accepting them and committing to meaningful actions based on the person's values. Ask yourself: "Is it my value to hate myself and to act on the emotions and behaviors that come from self-hatred?"

The Younger You

Imagine a young child coming to you, crying, telling you that they hate themselves. Do you have hatred for them, or do you want to take them in your arms and relieve them of their suffering? Do you have compassion for that child? What if that child is *you*? The idea of practicing compassion for a younger self—especially one who was hurt or devalued by others—centers on recognizing and nurturing the part of you that experienced pain, neglect, or unmet needs during childhood. To do this, there are several key principles:

- **Acknowledgment:** Healing begins by recognizing that the younger version of yourself carries the memories and emotions from the past, ones that have shaped your adult reactions today. Taking time to reflect on how those experiences molded your beliefs and personality is vital.
- **Validation and kindness:** Rather than dismissing or judging your younger self's pain, you recognize and acknowledge the experiences, reminding yourself that the hurt you experienced was real and undeserved. By providing yourself with the validation and care that you did not receive back then, you start to heal those old wounds.
- **Self-compassion practices:** This involves treating your younger self with the same kindness, reassurance, and support you would offer a loved friend or your own child. Practices can include visualizing comforting your younger self, writing letters of reassurance, or speaking kindly to that part of yourself.
- **Letting go of shame and blame:** Approaching your younger self with compassion allows you to let go of lingering shame, guilt, or self-blame that resulted from others' actions. It is a way of affirming that what happened was not your fault and that you are worthy of love and care. And, again, if

it helps, then visualize a young child being treated in the way you yourself were treated; you would never blame that child for what happened.

- **Fostering growth and resilience:** Nurturing the younger self fosters a capacity for self-validation that in turn can lead to greater self-acceptance, emotional resilience, and healthier coping mechanisms moving forward. Many of these are the skills we discuss throughout the book. As you practice compassion, you create a more authentic, and even safer, internal environment that supports emotional growth and greater peace with your history.

By regularly reminding yourself that who you are today was shaped by the experiences of a younger you, and doing so through these compassionate actions—providing comforting and caring—you deepen your relationship with yourself and gradually see the way these past experiences shaped you and that you are not to blame. The process is ongoing, but every act of self-kindness helps reinforce your inherent worth and supports lasting transformation.

Addressing Self-Hatred in Relationships

Self-hatred can severely impact relationships by shaping the way you perceive yourself and how you interact with others. Here are the major ways it affects connections with romantic partners, friends, and family:

- **Difficulty in accepting love:** Someone who intensely dislikes themselves may find it hard to believe they are lovable or worthy, leading to the rejection or mistrust of genuine affection from others. This creates tension, as the partner's positive view directly contradicts their negative self-image. Also, it is very confusing for the other person who may genuinely love you and yet this love is met with your skepticism.
- **Heightened sensitivity and jealousy:** Self-hatred often increases sensitivity to criticism—whether the criticism is real or perceived—and it can heighten the fear of abandonment or rejection. Even minor comments can be blown out of proportion, causing unnecessary conflict, jealousy, and emotional distance.
- **Withdrawal:** Believing that you are unworthy of love can drive behaviors such as withdrawal, pushing others away, or ending relationships prematurely out of fear that the other person will eventually leave anyway.

- **Overdependence or people-pleasing:** People struggling with self-hatred may seek constant validation or reassurance from friends and partners. They might become overly dependent on others, coming across as needy; have trouble setting boundaries; or prioritize others' needs to their own detriment, leading to resentment and imbalance in relationships. TIP: Doing the right thing for you, as long as it is within your values, is never doing the wrong thing for other people, and conversely, doing the wrong thing for you in order to please someone else is never doing the right thing for the other person.
- **Perpetuation of loneliness:** These patterns can reinforce social isolation, as the pain of expected rejection or criticism causes further withdrawal, making it difficult to maintain or form healthy, supportive connections.

Ultimately, self-hatred undermines intimacy, trust, communication, and satisfaction in all types of relationships. Healing often requires developing self-compassion and healthier self-worth to break these patterns and foster more positive, supportive bonds with others.

Values and Hope

In ACT, the focus of values and hope is central to guiding meaningful change and sustaining motivation.

Values in ACT are your deeply held personal principles and what truly matters to you in life. Identifying your values helps you define a clear direction and purpose. Living according to your values provides a framework for making choices and taking actions that bring fulfillment and a sense of meaning, even amid difficult thoughts or feelings.

Hope in the ACT context arises from the recognition that, while you cannot always control or eliminate painful emotions or challenging circumstances, you have the power to choose actions aligned with your values. This creates a hopeful outlook focused on growth, resilience, and a meaningful life beyond suffering.

When it comes to self-hatred, the focus on values and hope in ACT can help by providing a clear and positive direction that moves beyond the cycle of negative self-judgment. Here's how this helps:

- **Clarifying values:** An ACT focus can help you identify your most deeply held personal values—those that truly matter to you. For many people with self-hatred, kindness, connection, and integrity are important values. If these are values of yours, by connecting to them, you can start to see yourself not only through the lens of your pain but also through what you want to cultivate in your life, creating a more compassionate and balanced self-view.

- **Creating hope through meaningful action:** Hope in ACT arises through committed action toward these values, despite difficult thoughts or emotions—and clearly, the experience of self-hatred can be unbearable. Instead of trying to fight or eliminate self-hatred directly—which can be overwhelming—ACT encourages you to take small, meaningful steps aligned with your values, fostering a sense of progress, dignity, and self-worth.
- **Reducing fusion with negative self-views:** Self-hatred often involves fusion, meaning that you fuse with the concept of self-hatred. You identify tightly with harsh self-critical thoughts. ACT's values focus helps you create psychological flexibility, allowing you to see your thoughts as mental events rather than ultimate truths and to choose actions that reflect your values rather than the ways in which you might be beating up on yourself.
- **Building self-compassion and acceptance:** Living according to your values often encourages gentler and more compassionate self-treatment. As you focus on your kindness, integrity, and desire for true connection and move away from all the ideas that act against your values, you will experience a growing self-acceptance, which counterintuitively includes your imperfections, and this will reduce the intensity of self-hatred over time.

In essence, the focus on values and hope provides you a pathway to reconnect with what gives your life meaning and to cultivate a kinder, more purposeful relationship with yourself, gradually lessening self-hate through acceptance and committed, value-driven living.

Use the following activities with your therapist to guide you through identifying, observing, and challenging self-hatred as a pattern—not an identity. These activities are designed to integrate reflection, acceptance, and cognitive restructuring skills, as appropriate for each person's needs. Allow your therapist to support you as you build these skills, and revisit the questions as you make progress. Be sure to focus on the INSIGHT prompts to discuss your responses and reflect on them.

Activity 4.1: Addressing the Cycle of Self-Hatred

Review your answer to the warm-up activity in this workbook chapter and keep that in mind as you answer the following questions. If you have trouble, re-read your answers to the warm-up activity, then consider what someone who cares about you would say in response to hearing your description of self-hatred.

INSIGHT: When you recognize a thought that reflects self-hatred, after describing the thought, reflect. Ask yourself:

- Is this thought a true and complete description of who you are?

  ____

  ____

  ____

  ____

- Can you see it as just one perspective among many?

  ____

  ____

  ____

  ____

Activity 4.2: Thoughts → Emotions → Behaviors

Think of a recent time you experienced self-hatred. Fill in the chart to map the cycle.

Step	My Example
Negative thought	

(continued)

(continued)

Emotion felt

Behavior

Consequence

- How did your thought of self-hatred influence how you felt? What were your emotions?

- Did your lead to emotions lead to specific behaviors? What were these?

- Did your behaviors lead to other emotions? Did your behaviors lead to more thoughts? Is there a specific cycle or pattern that you can see?

____

____

____

____

- What was the outcome of the behavior—did it help or hurt in the long run?

____

____

____

____

INSIGHT: Can you identify any patterns? Write them down in the following diagram.

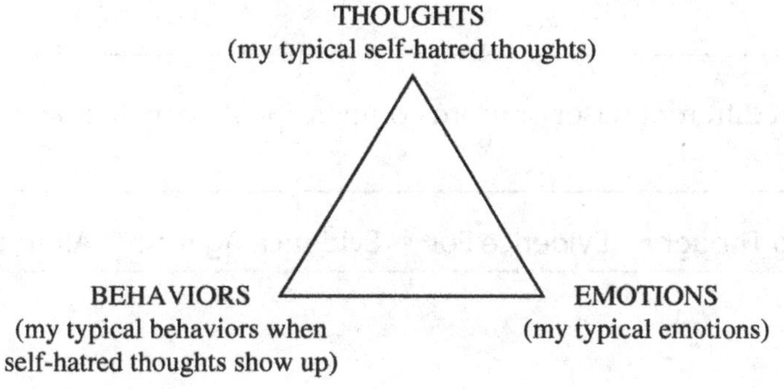

- What might you do differently if you notice this cycle starting again?

____

____

____

____

Activity 4.3: Challenging the Self-Hatred Narrative (CBT/ACT)

- Write down a recent self-hating thought. It could be as straightforward as "I hate myself" but can include variations such as "I hate myself because I . . ."

  ____

  ____

  ____

  ____

- Examine the evidence for and against this thought. What actual data do you have that supports the thought, beyond the fact that you have the thought?

  ____

  ____

  ____

  ____

- Is there a different wiser or more compassionate conclusion you could reach?

  ____

Self-Hating Thought	Evidence For	Evidence Against	Alternative Thought

INSIGHT: How does it feel to consider that your self-hatred might be based on old, unchallenged beliefs?

____

____

____

____

Activity 4.4: Self-Compassion for Your Younger Self (DBT/ACT)

Picture yourself as a child. If it helps, find a photo, or various photos, of younger you. Consider this person in your answers to the following questions:

- What would you say to this younger version of you if they expressed self-hatred? How would you listen to your younger self?

  ____

  ____

  ____

  ____

- Write a compassionate letter or message to your younger self.

  ____

  ____

  ____

  ____

INSIGHT: How does it feel to offer kindness to yourself, even if it's difficult?

____

____

____

____

Activity 4.5: Relationships and Trust (ACT/CBT)

Reflect on how self-hatred affects your relationships and answer the following questions:

- How has self-hatred impacted your relationships? Consider all relationships: romantic, family, work, friends, and so on.

  ____

  ____

  ____

  ____

- Do you believe others when they say positive things about you? Why or why not?

  ____

  ____

  ____

  ____

- What assumptions do you make about how others see you?

  ____

  ____

  ____

  ____

- List three examples of positive feedback you've received. What stops you from believing such feedback?

  ____

  ____

  ____

  ____

INSIGHT: Is it possible that others see strengths and value in you that you do not yet recognize?

____

____

____

____

Activity 4.6: Values and Hope (ACT)

Consider your values—the things that matter most to you—and begin to think about how you can pursue them to help you find hope. Remember that you can connect to your values by taking meaningful action. Even if you take small steps toward your values, you can improve your lived experience by connecting with the things that are most important to you.

The following questions will walk you through this process:

- Imagine a life without self-hatred. What would that look like? What would be possible for you?

  ____

  ____

  ____

  ____

- What values or dreams have you put aside because of self-hatred?

  ____

  ____

  ____

  ____

- List one small step you could take toward a value or goal, even if self-hatred is present.

____

____

____

____

INSIGHT: What does it mean to move toward hope, even if you still struggle with self-hatred?

____

____

____

____

Key Points

- Self-hatred creates a harmful cycle where negative thoughts lead to painful emotions, which drive behaviors that reinforce the negative beliefs.
- People with self-hatred have difficult relationships because they struggle to accept love, experience heightened sensitivity, and may engage in people-pleasing or withdrawal.
- ACT can offer a pathway to break free by focusing on meaningful action aligned with personal values rather than fighting self-hatred directly.
- Practicing compassion for one's younger self can help heal childhood wounds and recognize that past pain was undeserved.
- Psychological flexibility allows adaptation beyond rigid patterns, while acknowledging and describing self-hatred helps create distance from it.

Chapter 5

What Is the Self That You Are Hating?

Chapter Summary

This chapter takes a philosophical turn to explore the root causes of self-hatred. If everything has a cause, and every causal factor also has a cause, it takes a lot of digging to understand anything on a deep level. Acknowledging this expands the scope of a person's considerations of why they feel self-loathing, and who or what is to blame. The root causes of self-hatred are not simple to uncover and, indeed, a person can continue looking backwards to find causes of causes of causes. This can be a helpful reminder that there is no single, identifiable cause for someone's self-loathing or negative thought patterns.

While some people with self-hatred also experience body dysmorphia and eating disorders (see Chapter 9), many believe that they would continue to hate themselves even if their body were replaced or eliminated. For most people, self-loathing is faulty conclusion generated by their thoughts, and those same thoughts perpetuate their negative feelings. Despite their extreme negative emotions, most people's bodies are doing everything they can to stay alive. Their hearts are pumping blood, their lungs are taking in oxygen, their nervous system is sending sensory signals, their kidneys are filtering their blood, their stomach is digesting food, and yet we do not hate our hearts, our lungs, our kidneys or stomach. These functions all continue, and are controlled to a lesser or greater extent by the brain despite that very same brain telling them that they are undeserving.

Now because we all have different brains, different experiences, different biology, and different development, even people looking at the exact same thing can interpret it differently. But different interpretations do not change the actual facts or chain of events. Yet interpretations of these facts and events can cause a lot of psychological damage. It doesn't change the lived experience of the person who is being perceived. But it can be helpful to remember that there are always many perspectives on something. Fables like "The Couple and the Donkey" (*I Hate Myself*, Chapter 5) can help a person with self-hatred recognize that other people may have different points of view. Even though someone feels certain that they are unworthy of love, support, care, success, or admiration, they may be willing to admit that other people may feel differently about them.

Key Definitions and Concepts

- **Invalidation:** The communication of messages that dismiss, minimize, or reject another person's thoughts, feelings, experiences, or perceptions.
- **Point of view:** The perspective from which a story is told or understood. A person's point of view is influenced by their individual experiences, and it shades their interpretation of the things they observe.
- **Root cause:** The core issue that drives a particular outcome. There is not a single root cause of human behavior because it emerges from complex interactions between multiple factors.

Rather than attempting to pinpoint the root cause of a person's self-loathing, it can be helpful to be willing to accept that it is a combination of factors, stretching through time, relationships, and experiences. It is also helpful to consider their point of view and recognize that their experience is not fixed or universal. Other people likely have very different opinions about a person with self-hatred; In fact, others often feel tremendous compassion for the person with self-loathing. Understanding this can encourage a person to focus on changing their immediate thoughts and behaviors, which is a far more productive approach than trying to answer the question *Why am I like this?*

Chapter 5 Warmup Activity

The thought "I hate myself" is just that—a thought, not a fact. How would you define the experience of self-hatred if you had to break down the thought in a descriptive way, including all its elements. How would you explain what you are experiencing to others? Use this worksheet to break down and describe this thought in detail by answering the following questions:

1. What does "I hate myself" mean to you? This is an open-ended question. Over the course of this workbook, you and your therapist should revisit this question over and over.

____

____

____

____

Theories of Self-Hatred and Therapeutic Approaches

Different psychological models have different theories of self-hatred. Understanding them can help you and your therapist identify the models and tools that will be most helpful in addressing your self-hatred. Cognitive behavioral therapy (CBT), dialectical behavioral therapy (DBT), and acceptance and commitment therapy (ACT) interact with these theories in different ways, and at times in overlapping ways.

Here is a summary of four major models:

- **Attitudinal stance and shame (CBT):** Attitudinal stance—the way a person relates to their own experience (judgmental versus curious, harsh versus compassionate, fused versus observing)—is a major amplifier or reducer of self-hatred. A hostile, fused stance turns painful experiences into evidence of being "bad," whereas a mindful, compassionate, decentered stance interrupts that conversion and allows pain without the added layer of self-loathing This theory uses CBT techniques to address shame by examining a person's attitudes and beliefs that produce shameful feelings. This often involves replacing distorted thinking patterns with more compassionate ones to improve a person's perception of themselves.
- **Model (CBT/ACT):** Self-disgust intensifies self-hatred by evoking visceral revulsion toward one's body, actions, or core self, often as a more embodied and isolating form of self-rejection compared to the more abstract self-hatred, leading to avoidance, self-harm urges, and entrenched shame. This model uses CBT or ACT techniques to help someone address intrusive thoughts related to self-disgust. CBT helps them replace these negative

thought patterns, while ACT encourages them to accept these thoughts while reducing their power.

- **Biosocial model (DBT):** DBT's biosocial model explains self-hatred and self-disgust in BPD as outcomes of a transaction between a biologically sensitive person and chronic invalidation, an interaction which amplifies shame-prone emotions into pervasive dysregulation and self-attack. This model uses DBT to explore invalidation (discussed in the next section) and the joint role of social and biological factors in a person's emotional response to it. By identifying the relationships, interactions, and circumstances that trigger self-hatred, and acknowledging the biological factors that contribute to it, someone can improve their emotional regulation during triggering situations.
- **Psychodynamic model:** The psychodynamic theory views self-hatred as arising from harsh superego formation, Superego formation is the process where a child absorbs parental and societal rules about right and wrong, creating an inner "moral voice" or conscience that guides behavior through guilt or pride. In this context, self-hatred arises when internalized parental criticism and having conflicted feelings toward loved people causes the person to turn their aggression inward leading to self-attacks and self-punishment. This model addresses unresolved conflicts, repressed emotions, and past experiences that contribute to self-hating thoughts. Working with a therapist, a person can work through these experiences and relationships, limiting their influence on the person's thoughts and behaviors.

Invalidation

When you experience invalidation, it is the communication that your thoughts, feelings, and behaviors are wrong, unacceptable, or don't make sense. The invalidating environment dismisses the experiences of your mind, at times punishing you for being you. Invalidation can include the following:

- Physical, emotional, and sexual abuse.
- Being compared to others whose behavior is considered more "appropriate."

- Being told that you are too much.
- Being told that you are not trying hard enough, or making it seem as if life's problems are easy to solve.

Think about the times that you were told that you were overreacting? You were simply reacting the way you did. Others may have judged you by comparing you to others and concluding that your reactions were more excessive than those of others. But just because you might have big reactions does not mean that you are either a bad person, wrong, or flawed. Imagine two people, one allergic to peanuts and the other not. Both eat a peanut. One has a big reaction and the other has none. Both are simply responding to eating a peanut. Neither is right nor wrong. To the highly sensitive person, certain interactions trigger a strong and often painful emotion. Being told not to respond the way you do is invalidating. Invalidation is painful, but it is not a teaching method. The fact that you have been invalidated does not mean that you have to believe the lessons of the invalidation.

However, having big and painful reactions to events, whether to a peanut or some emotional event, can have serious consequences. It is possible to learn and adapt so you can more effectively deal with things that trigger you. This allows you to develop more agency and self-advocacy.

Invalidation can show you that other people may have been instrumental in the way you see yourself, but blaming them won't help you get out of the cycle of self-hatred. Once you understand the potential impact of invalidation, and the role it has played in your life, you can help yourself heal.

In most circumstances, the people invalidating you did not know about invalidation and its impact. Your parents likely were doing the best they could, and used methods that they expected to work, or that did work with other siblings. Sensitive people respond very deeply to invalidation, even if for others it has few consequences.

The following activities integrate psychoeducation, reflection, and evidence-based therapeutic strategies. They are designed to help you and your therapist explore the origins of your self-hatred and understand how your early experiences and invalidation shaped your self-concept. Then, you will use your evolving understanding to develop a new and kinder way of treating yourself. Activities 5.1 through 5.3 focus on the roots of your self-hatred and which theories are the best fit for your specific experience. In Activities 5.4 through 5.7, you will use tools from some of the different types of therapies to begin to expand your awareness of the various elements of your early childhood as a way to make self-hatred less of an abstract thought.

Activity 5.1: Mapping the Timeline of Self-Hatred

For most people who are reading this book, the seeds of self-hatred were planted early in childhood, and the roots began to take hold in a mind that was fertile to believe its toxicity. Recognizing that you were not born with self-hatred, but that you learned to hate yourself because you were taught to hate yourself, is an important step in healing from its grip.

Reflect on your earliest memories of self-loathing or any unhealthy and unhelpful self-evaluation. Use the prompts below to help map your timeline.

- How far back do you remember feeling self-loathing or self-judgment?

____

____

____

____

- What specific thoughts and emotions do you remember?

____

____

____

____

- What was happening in your life at that time?

____

____

____

____

- Were there specific events, messages, or comparisons that stand out?

- Can you recall a time before these feelings began? What was different?

Use the following table to organize your thoughts about past events that were invalidating, traumatic, or contributed to your negative feelings in some other way.

Age/Period	Memory/Event	Associated Feelings/Thoughts

(continued)

(continued)

Activity 5.2: Exploring the Roots—Reflection Prompts

Choose one or more prompts to write about or discuss with your therapist.

- What early experiences, family dynamics, or social situations contributed to your sense of being "bad," "unlovable," or "flawed"?

- Were there times you were compared, as being less than, to others (for example, a sibling at home or other child in school) or blamed for things that were outside of your control?

____

____

____

____

- Did you experience invalidation (e.g., feelings dismissed, told you were "too sensitive," or "overreacting")?

____

____

____

____

- How did you cope with these experiences as a child?

____

____

____

____

- What would you tell your younger self if you met them today?

____

____

____

____

In this next exercise you will review the theoretical underpinnings of self-hatred.

Activity 5.3: Theories of Self-Hatred—Psychoeducation and Personal Application

Review the brief descriptions of each theory below. For each, note whether it applies to your experience and, if so, how.

Theory/Model	Summary Description	Does This Fit My Experience? How?
Attitudinal stance & shame (CBT)	Negative self-beliefs + self-criticism leading to shame and self-punishment	
Disgust model (CBT/ACT)	Wanting to distance yourself from "disgusting" parts of self, often after trauma	
Biosocial model (DBT)	Being a highly sensitive person + invalidating environment leading to chronic shame/ self-hatred	
Psychodynamic model	Early unmet needs, attachment wounds, and unconscious conflict shape your self-concept	

Activity 5.4: Awareness of Invalidation (DBT/Mindfulness)

In this activity, focus on nonfamilial relationships, for instance, teachers, coaches, religious people, kids, neighbors, and any other people who impacted your sense of self.

Recall times when your feelings or experiences were dismissed, minimized, or punished.

- Who were the main people involved?

- Are these people still in your life?

- What messages did you receive then about your emotions or needs?

- Are you still receiving these messages today?

- How did you respond at the time?

- If you are still being invalidated, how do you respond now?

- Can you recognize how the enduring invalidation shaped your beliefs about yourself?

____

____

____

____

- Where there any people in your life who were validating, who did protect you, who saw the possibility in you?

____

____

____

____

Now moving on to your family, including parents, siblings and extended family.

Activity 5.5: Family Comparison and Sibling Dynamics

Reflect on your family environment.

- Who was in your family in your early childhood, and which extended family members did you have regular contact with?

____

____

____

____

- Did you feel you had to be "the perfect child" or that you were "the problem"?

____

____

____

____

- If so, what were the specific messages that led you to believe this?

- If you have siblings or cousins, were you compared to them?

- What were the specific comparisons and how did these affect your self-view?

- Did you feel that you were treated differently?

- If so, how did your caregivers respond differently to you and others?

Now reflect on the experiences in Activities 5.4 and 5.5 as you consider the next set of exercises.

Activity 5.6: Internalization and Shame (CBT/ACT)

Identify beliefs or messages you internalized from early experiences. Internalization is the process of taking in external ideas, values, rules, or attitudes from others (like parents or society) and making them your own inner beliefs or motivations, so they guide your thoughts and actions automatically.

- What are some core beliefs you hold about yourself today that originated in childhood?

  ____

  ____

  ____

  ____

- How do these beliefs affect your current emotions and behaviors?

  ____

  ____

  ____

  ____

- How do they affect everyday interactions with the people in your life, at work, at school, in your faith or social community?

  ____

  ____

  ____

  ____

- How do they affect your family relationships?

  ____

  ____

  ____

  ____

- Where there any positive messages that you received, even if you didn't completely believe them?

___

___

___

___

- If you were to believe that the people who expressed these more compassionate messages were being honest, are there ways now that you could incorporate those elements in how you see yourself?

___

___

___

___

The work of breaking the cycle of self-hatred involves the repeated practice of focusing on and eroding its patterns, recognizing that it was learned, and then developing kinder ways of treating yourself.

Activity 5.7: Step-by-Step Mapping Exercise (DBT/ACT)

Before starting this activity, you need to understand the concept of reinforcement. Reinforcement is any consequence that occurs after a behavior that makes it more likely that the behavior will happen again in the future. Unhealthy behaviors are reinforcing because they provide temporary relief from negative emotions or achieve perceived benefits, creating a cycle where the behavior offers a short-term solution to overwhelming stress, anxiety, or self-criticism. For instance, with the behavior of self-injury, this relief can come from a reduction in emotional pain, while for the behavior of perfectionism, it might stem from the temporary soothing of fears of failure and self-blame associated with perceived mistakes. Over time, these behaviors can become conditioned responses, becoming automatic habits that are difficult to change even when they are harmful.

Map out how your self-hatred developed, step by step.

Step	My Experience/Example
Biological predisposition (e.g., family history, sensitivity)	
Invalidation (e.g., specific invalidating events or messages)	
Acceptance-seeking (e.g., trying to please/calm others, fear-based behaviors)	
More invalidation (e.g., repeated dismissal or blame)	
Internalization (e.g., starting to believe it's your fault)	
Shame (e.g., feeling fundamentally flawed)	
Reinforced behaviors (e.g., self-harm, avoidance, perfectionism)	
Self-hatred (e.g., core beliefs, identity statements)	

Key Points

- Self-hatred has complex, multiple root causes that cut across time, relationships, and experiences. There is no single identifiable source.
- Invalidation (dismissal of thoughts, feelings, and experiences) plays a major role in developing self-hatred, especially for sensitive individuals.
- Other people's perspectives on you are often far more compassionate than your own, highlighting that self-hatred is not a universal truth.
- Recognizing that self-hatred was learned rather than innate is crucial for beginning the healing process.

Part 2

Roots of Self-Hatred

Understanding the roots of self-hatred is important because it will help you recognize that it is not an intrinsic part of you. You are not destined to live with self-loathing. You have the power to change your negative thoughts, and you don't need to do it alone. This workbook, *I Hate Myself,* and your therapist are here to support you. The Part 2 Activity is designed to help you take the first step toward change and remind you that there are people in your life who care for you and want to support you.

Part 2 Activity: Taking the First Step Toward Change

Identify one belief or behavior related to self-hatred that you're willing to question or challenge this week.

1. What small act of self-kindness can you try, even if it feels uncomfortable?

    ____

    ____

    ____

    ____

2. Other than your therapist, who else can you ask for support as you begin this work?

    ____

    ____

    ____

    ____

Chapter 6

Where Does Self-Hatred Come From?

Chapter Summary

People aren't born with any kind of hatred, including hatred of the self. While some people don't have any memories of their lives before self-hatred, this doesn't mean it is an innate part of anyone. It's something that's learned, typically during early childhood or adolescence. Few people can pinpoint a single experience that caused them to hate themselves, which can lead people to believe that they were born hating themselves. In reality, these feelings develop gradually and become stronger with time.

People I've worked with typically recall first experiencing self-hatred after recognizing that they struggled with something, like anxiety, difficulty socializing with peers, a sense they were disappointing people, or envy of others who went through life apparently without these problems. This led many of them to draw the conclusion that, not only was there something wrong with them, but that they were also responsible for their pervasive thoughts and behaviors. This can generate the negative thinking patterns that reinforce self-hatred, making it feel like an integral part of a person over time.

The good news is that self-hatred can be unlearned, and mindfulness is a key tool. This chapter offers specific exercises and techniques to show that self-loathing is not an intrinsic or necessary part of anyone's being. For example, one exercise has readers look at photos of themselves at every age and really consider whether it's possible for them to hate the child in those photos. This helps a person expand their idea of the self and realize that they can unlearn self-hatred and cultivate self-compassion.

Four Key Theories

Chapter 6 of *I Hate Myself* covers four theories related to self-hatred and how to apply each one to help unlearn self-hatred. Here is a review of them:

1. **Roy Krawitz's attitudinal emotional stance:** A person's attitude about something they think or do combines with shame, self-criticism, and negative self-judgment. Over time, a negative attitudinal emotional stance can lead to self-hatred. *Application*: Practice alternate responses to shame, self-criticism, and negative self-judgment so you can replace them and develop a new attitudinal emotional stance that supports resilience and a healthier self-image.
2. **Rottraut Ille's self-disgust theory:** People with self-hatred are repelled by aspects of themselves and believe they are permanently flawed and unredeemable. This is common among people who have had traumatic experiences like abuse and cannot separate themselves from that experience. *Application*: Acknowledging the reasons for your self-disgust with your therapist (or another qualified, trustworthy person) can help you recognize that you did not deserve your traumatic experiences and should not let them define you.
3. **Marsha Linehan's biosocial model (DBT):** Chronic emotional dysregulation emerges when a child is repeatedly invalidated (see Chapter 5). Newborns have an innate capacity to attract the care they need for survival, and as children grow, they need more emotional support. These needs vary from person to person, and someone with stronger needs may feel rejected or unworthy of care. *Application*: Family systems therapy can attempt to change this dynamic so the environment responds more supportively to a person's needs. Individually, a person can analyze the role of invalidation in their feelings of self-loathing. This can help them understand that the self-loathing is not innate; rather, it's an emotional response to their environment. Then, they can work on ways to seek the support they need and develop resilience.
4. **Psychodynamic model in borderline personality disorder:** A person's early life experiences cause their longstanding beliefs and desires. This happens on an unconscious level. Self-hatred emerges as a maladaptive way of coping with negative life experiences that a person hasn't yet processed. This can result in a person struggling to integrate seemingly separate parts of themselves into a whole that makes sense. In this model, a person's

self-hatred is a symptom of attachment disorder. *Application*: By addressing the struggle between the wanted and rejected self, you can unpack your childhood trauma and learn how to develop kinder feelings for yourself.

Key Definitions and Concepts

- **Self-talk:** A person's internal dialogue or stream of thoughts. Positive or negative, it influences their emotions, behaviors, and self-perception.
- **Attitudinal emotional stance:** A person's beliefs about their actions, thoughts, and behaviors, combined with the emotions they generate, and how that influences their self-concept and identity.
- **Biosocial model:** A way of understanding emotions and behaviors that focuses on the transaction between a person's biology and their environment.
- **Psychodynamic model:** A way of understanding self-hatred and borderline personality disorder as maladaptive ways of coping with unresolved childhood trauma.
- **Mindfulness:** The practice of paying attention, with purpose, to the present moment and viewing it without judgment.
- **Cognitive defusion:** Separating thoughts and facts to reduce the emotional power of negative thoughts and recognize that they are not necessarily true.

Ultimately, where self-hatred comes from isn't the point of therapy. The goal is to understand that your self-hatred is rooted in childhood experiences; it is not a choice or an innate part of who you are. By having compassion for your childhood self, you can begin to undo the damage created by their harmful experiences. If you feel that some of these exercises are repetitive, it is because they are! It is important to remember that self-hatred is learned, and you need multiple repetitions of healthy reflection to unlearn the false teachings.

Chapter 6 Warmup Activity: Case Example Reflection

You are not alone in your experience of self-hatred. Many others have gone through similar incidents, and this activity can help you to join the community of those who have struggled as you have. You are not alone, even if it feels that way, and working through these exercises can remind you of that.

Read the following account, which is taken from *I Hate Myself*.

> *During the period of diagnosis and worsening of my physical health, my self-hatred changed and increased significantly due to the phenomena described above. I felt that my body was annoying, defective, useless, and a burden to my family and society. This, in combination with the way my disability affected my social life and sense of belongingness as a child, has had a significant effect on my self-hatred, suicidality, and use of maladaptive coping skills, such as self-harm and eating disorder behaviors.*

- What stands out to you in this story?

____

____

____

____

- Can you relate to any part of this experience?

____

____

____

____

- How has your own health, disability, or sense of difference affected your self-view?

____

____

____

____

- Can you have compassion for the person who wrote those words. If they were someone important in your life, what would you say to them?

____

____

____

____

Strategies for Reducing Self-Hatred

Given that the narrative of self-hatred can be so deeply entrenched, challenging it is hard, and even harder if you don't believe that it can change. There are some specific strategies taught in acceptance and commitment therapy (ACT) that can help.

Cognitive defusion: Notice self-critical thoughts as just thoughts, not facts. Defusion is the opposite of fusion. Fusion is fusing your thoughts, that are just thoughts, as facts. Defusion is separating thoughts, that are just thoughts, from facts. One way to practice this, for example, is hearing your inner critic saying things like, "You are not good enough" and responding by saying something like, "There you go again, mind" or picturing the thought as if it were a leaf floating away on a river current. Other defusion techniques include practices such as repeating negative statements in a silly voice or as a song, which helps reduce their emotional power and make them less believable. It is almost as if you were teasing your mind for being ridiculous for having the thoughts you are having.

Values clarification and committed action: The idea here is to shift your focus from battling negative thoughts to acting according to personal values, such as kindness, courage, or integrity. Ask yourself if your inner critic's message is consistent with your values. If not, gently set it aside and choose actions that move toward what matters most, even in the presence of self-critical thoughts.

Next is to work on reducing burdensomeness by building connection, and again we can turn to ACT, which reduces the feeling of burdensomeness by helping you shift attention away from negative self-evaluations including self-hatred and toward meaningful connection, openness, and value-driven action in relationships. Again, you can use a practice like defusion. For example, labeling the thought ("I notice I'm having the thought that I'm a burden") creates distance from thought and "fact" and reduces its impact on self-hatred. ACT also encourage you to reach out, initiate connection, and participate in meaningful activities aligned with your values. This may mean that you initially have to give up friendships that have not shared your values and find new connections.

The Role of Mindfulness

Mindfulness is the core skill of DBT and a central concept in ACT. It is the practice of observing the present moment without judging it and noting all its elements. Being able to notice the present moment in its entirety allows for greater control of the experience. Here's a simple example of its application. Make yourself a cup of tea or coffee, or any other drink you want. How often do you sit and savor the drink—its smell, it taste, its temperature? How often are you doing something else when you drink? Drinking while scrolling on social media, watching TV, driving in your car, speaking to someone else. I happen to love Earl Grey tea. Drinking a cup of freshly brewed tea, knowing that I am drinking it, smelling it, savoring it, is a very different experience to not being present with it.

However, it is one thing drinking your favorite cup of tea, but what happens when in the present moment, there is a lot of negativity, and your brain is flooded with painful emotions and unwanted thoughts? For people in therapy who are struggling with such experiences, mindfulness can be difficult for the following reasons:

- **Emotional intensity:** Painful emotions like grief, fear, anger, or deep sadness may arise with such force that it feels intolerable to sit with them and observe them. The mind instinctively seeks to avoid this discomfort, making it challenging to stay present.
- **Habitual avoidance:** Many people are conditioned to cope with pain by distracting, suppressing, or pushing away difficult feelings. Mindfulness asks us to do the opposite—turn toward discomfort—which can feel unnatural and even frightening at first.
- **Fear of being overwhelmed:** There can be a worry that paying attention to painful thoughts or emotions will make them worse or that they will spiral out of control. This fear can make mindful awareness feel risky.
- **Negative self-judgment:** People may judge themselves for having painful emotions or believe such feelings are signs of weakness or failure, leading to resistance against acknowledging them with mindful awareness.
- **Physical discomfort:** Painful thoughts and emotions often trigger uncomfortable physical sensations (tightness, agitation, heaviness), making it even harder to remain present.

Despite these challenges, practicing mindfulness gently and with compassionate curiosity can help you gradually build tolerance for discomfort, reframe your relationship with pain, and ultimately foster acceptance and healing. The key is to approach these experiences with non-judgment and kindness, taking breaks as needed, and recognizing that it's okay if mindfulness feels hard sometimes. Also, when a painful memory arises, the ability to be present with that memory allows you to label that as an experience of the past, and not one that is happening right now. It is quite different to have a memory of drinking a cup than to be drinking a cup of tea.

The practice of mindfulness can significantly reduce self-hatred by transforming the way you relate to your thoughts and feelings:

- **Creates a pause:** Mindfulness teaches you to notice self-critical thoughts as they arise, creating a pause before you react emotionally or believe them. This pause helps you recognize that such thoughts are your brain creating a story that is different from the facts of who you are, making it easier to observe them with curiosity rather than judgment.
- **Fosters self-compassion:** Self-compassion can be an aversive concept for people tackling self-hatred, and yet it is the ultimate destination. By repeatedly practicing non-judgmental awareness, mindfulness cultivates a kinder, more compassionate inner voice. Instead of harsh self-criticism, you learn to treat yourself with warmth and understanding during difficult moments, eventually breaking the cycle of self-loathing.
- **Reduces identification with negative self-talk:** Mindfulness allows you to see negative self-talk as passing mental chatter, a part of the thousands of thoughts that pass through your brain every day, rather than absolute truth. This helps diminish its emotional impact, helping create greater emotional balance and self-acceptance over time.
- **Improves self-worth:** Practicing mindfulness can directly and temporarily boost self-esteem, as it helps you stay present rather than ruminating on perceived failures or inadequacies. Even if you think you are a terrible person, in this moment as you read this sentence, surely there have been times you have felt worse about yourself. You are not such a terrible person right now, and by the time you do all the exercises in this book, you will see how incredible you are.

Through regular mindfulness practice, you gradually weaken the grip of self-hatred, nurture a sense of self-worth, and lay the foundation for ongoing emotional healing and well-being.

The following activities will help you and your therapist practice what is described in this chapter, so you can understand the interplay of psychological and biological factors. You will also target key vulnerability factors such as perceived burdensomeness and failed belongingness, which can drive suicidal thinking and behavior.

Activity 6.1: Challenging the Narrative (CBT/ACT)

Identify a self-hating thought related to being a burden or not belonging.

- What is the evidence for and against this thought?

____

____

____

____

- If there is no factual evidence, have you fused your thought with "facts" and made your thought a fact?

____

____

____

____

- Can you defuse your thought by saying something like "mind, you created an unhelpful thought, and I am choosing a more compassionate thought"?

____

____

____

____

- Is there another way to view your role in relationships or your community?

____

____

____

____

- Label thoughts as thoughts and label facts as facts. For instance: *I am having the thought that I hate myself*, which might be tied to the fact that you arrived 30 minutes late to work.

- Can you defuse the thought and the fact? "The fact that I arrived 30 minutes late to work led to the thought that *I hate myself*. While the fact is a fact, the thought is not."

Activity 6.2: Building Connection and Reducing Burdensomeness (DBT/ACT)

- List three ways you contribute to the lives of others, no matter how small the contribution.

  1.

  2.

  3.

- Identify one person or group where you feel even a small sense of belonging.

- Write down the names of the people in your life and how they act in the world, and then ask yourself if their values are consistent with yours. Explain how or how not.

____

____

____

____

- If your group does not share your values, is there a way to accept the sadness and disappointment of your situation, and then consider other people in your life who you might not have connected with for whatever reason, who are worth trying to get to know?

____

____

____

____

- What is one action you could take this week to strengthen a sense of connection?

____

____

____

____

Activity 6.3: Mindfulness of Thoughts (Mindfulness/DBT/ACT)

Practice observing your self-hating thoughts as just thoughts—not facts; then answer the insight question.

- Sit quietly and notice when the thought "I hate myself" arises.
- Label it as "just a thought."
- Keep on noticing it until it passes. (One practice that has helped some of my clients is to lie in a park on a sunny day and find a cloud that they label

the cloud of self-hate. They watch it as it dissolves, and sometimes it gets bigger, but it always changes and eventually it disappears. Thoughts, like clouds and life itself, are always in transformation.)

Optional Practices:

- Imagine sitting in front of a loved one and telling them that you hate yourself.
- Repeat the thought out loud until it loses its emotional charge.
- Write the thought down, then shred the paper, or write it on toilet paper and flush it down the toilet.

INSIGHT: What happens when you observe your thoughts without judgment or attachment?

____

____

____

____

Activity 6.4: Compassionate Self-Talk

Many people with self-hatred find the idea of compassionate self-talk to be pointless, not applicable to them, or self-invalidating. There are two approaches that might challenge this obstacle to more self-compassion.

1. **A friend:** Imagine a friend is struggling with the same feelings of self-hatred. What would you say to them?

   ____

   ____

   ____

   ____

   Now, write a message of kindness to yourself.

   ____

   ____

   ____

   ____

2. **Your younger self:** Imagine yourself as the young child who was criticized, bullied, or mistreated—the one who learned to believe that they were flawed. Write down what you would say to that child if they were with you now.

____

____

____

____

Key Points

- Self-hatred is learned and develops gradually through childhood experiences of struggle, disappointment, and perceived failure.
- Four key theories explain origins: attitudinal emotional stance (shame + negative attitudes), self-disgust theory (feeling permanently flawed), the biosocial model (invalidation + emotional needs), and the psychodynamic model (unprocessed childhood trauma).
- Mindfulness practice helps create distance from self-hating thoughts by observing them without judgment as transient mental events.
- Cognitive defusion techniques (like labeling thoughts as "just thoughts" or using a silly voice) reduce the emotional power of self-criticism.
- Connecting with a younger self and showing that child compassion can help unlearn harmful messages from childhood.

Chapter 7

Could It Be Temperament or Biology?

Chapter Summary

No research demonstrates self-hatred has a genetic or temperamental component, but one study hints at the possibility that it could have genetic or biological risk factors. This chapter discusses the topic of suicide, so I will repeat the trigger warning that is in Chapter 7 of *I Hate Myself*: SUICIDE IS NOT THE ANSWER. Reading personal accounts of suicidal ideation can bring these thoughts to the front of someone's mind when they are struggling with self-hatred or other mental health conditions. If you have thoughts of suicide, please immediately contact someone you trust. If you have a therapist, counselor, or other professional helping you with self-hatred, you can contact them as well.

Some research shows that genetics strongly influences suicidal behavior (40–50 percent), and psychological and environmental factors account for 50–60 percent of suicidal behavior. The Interpersonal-Psychological Theory of Suicide (IPTS) outlines the risk factors:

1. Perceived burdensomeness
2. Failed belongingness
3. The acquired capability for suicide

Additionally, IPTS states that for someone to die by suicide, they have to desire suicide. Strong genetic components that factor into this desire are pain tolerance and not being afraid of death. To reduce suicide risk, therapy should focus on perceived burdensomeness and failed belongingness because these are more likely to change with appropriate therapeutic interventions.

Physical pain also has links to suicidal behavior. For example, people who experience chronic pain are twice as likely to make a suicide attempt as people who do not have chronic pain. Patients who self-injure and don't feel pain also have a higher risk of suicidal behaviors. In these patients, not being afraid of pain increases their likelihood of suicide. By contrast, many other people are afraid of the expected pain, and that prevents them from making a suicide attempt.

Key Definitions and Concepts

- **Interpersonal-Psychological Theory of Suicide (IPTS):** The main theory to explain why people die by suicide.
- **Thwarted belongingness:** Feelings of disconnection or alienation.
- **Perceived burdensomeness:** The belief that a person must be cared for or tolerated by others and has nothing positive to offer.
- **Acquired capability for suicide:** The combination of having a low fear of death and a high pain tolerance.
- **Hopelessness:** The belief that nothing will get better.

If you feel that some of these exercises are repetitive, it is because they are! It is important to remember that self-hatred is learned, and you need multiple repetitions of healthy reflection to unlearn the false teachings.

Chapter 7 Warmup Activity: Mapping the Sources of My Self-Hatred

This is a review of the different factors that contributed to your self-hatred and is similar to the exercise you did in Chapter 5. For each category below, write down memories, experiences, or patterns that stand out.

Source/Factor	My Experience/Example
Family environment	

Source/Factor	My Experience/Example
School/social experiences	
Chronic illness/pain	
Genetics/biology	
Cultural messages	
Other	

Interpersonal-Psychological Theory of Suicide (IPTS)

This chapter dives deeper into the origins of self-hatred, exploring various elements including the roles of environmental, biological, and temperamental factors as well as the impact of certain conditions, such as depression, anxiety, and chronic pain.

First, let's review the Interpersonal-Psychological Theory of Suicide (IPTS), which is a prevailing theory that attempts to explain why people die by suicide.

It identifies three key psychological constructs: thwarted belongingness, perceived burdensomeness, and acquired capability for suicide.

Here is a deeper dive into these core constructs:

- **Perceived burdensomeness:** This is the belief that you are a burden to others or society, and that loved ones would be better off if you were gone because you feel that all you do is cause them trouble.
- **Thwarted belongingness:** This is the feeling of being isolated, lonely, or that you do not belong to any significant group or relationship.
- **Acquired capability for suicide:** This is the gradual development of a reduced fear of death and an increased tolerance for physical pain. This typically develops through repeated exposure to painful or fear-inducing situations (such as self-injury, trauma, or abuse).

A fourth concept that is not core to the IPTS but significant nonetheless is that of hopelessness. Hopelessness is the sense that things will never get better, which in the context of self-hatred adds to the burden because of the certainty that it will never change. Table 7.1 outlines these constructs and their role in suicide risk.

Next, let's look at the impact of physical and emotional pain, and you will see how this ties to the concepts you have just reviewed. First, chronic physical and/or emotional pain can shape self-hatred and risk for self-injury and suicidal thinking. Continuous pain—whether physical or emotional—can limit

Table 7.1 Core Constructs of IPTS

Construct	Description	Role in Suicide Risk
Thwarted belongingness	Feeling disconnected or alienated	Contributes to desire for suicide
Perceived burdensomeness	Belief of being a burden	Contributes to desire for suicide
Acquired capability	Low fear of death, high pain tolerance	Enables suicide attempt
Hopelessness	Belief that states won't improve	Intensifies risk and ideation

your ability to engage in daily activities, maintain relationships, and pursue goals, leading to diminished self-worth and a sense of inadequacy. Over time, these limitations and perceived failures can foster excessive self-criticism and then aggravate your feelings of being a burden, reinforcing beliefs of unworthiness. Then, chronic pain might force you to withdraw socially, because either it is too painful to do anything, it is too painful to enjoy yourself, or the unpredictability of when pain might surge can lead to worsening feelings of loneliness and exclusion. This isolation not only amplifies emotional suffering but also diminishes access to supportive feedback, making negative self-talk more dominant and deepening your sense of being flawed and which can aggravate your self-hatred.

Finally, here is a mindfulness practice to help with pain which comes from a particular form of mindfulness therapy known as Mindfulness-Based Stress Reduction (MBSR). It typically involves an eight-week course with group sessions using meditation, gentle movement (yoga), and guided mindfulness exercises that train attentional focus and acceptance.

Position and intention

- Lie down or sit in a supported position where your body is relatively still but awake.
- Set the frame: "The goal is not to make my pain disappear, but to explore it with curiosity and kindness."

Anchoring attention

- Begin with a few minutes of awareness of the breath in the abdomen or chest, just noticing the rise and fall.
- When attention wanders, gently note "thinking" or "drifting" and come back to the breath.

Systematic body scan

- Move your attention slowly and sequentially through the body (e.g., toes → feet → calves → knees → thighs → pelvis → abdomen → chest → hands → arms → shoulders → neck → face → scalp).
- In each region, notice sensations: pressure, pulsing, heat, cold, tingling, numbness, or pain—whatever is there—without judging it as good or bad.

If a region is painful, linger for a few breaths:

Name it softly ("tightness," "burning," "stabbing," "pulling").

Notice its size, shape, edges, intensity, and whether it shifts from moment to moment.

"Allowing" and widening

Instead of tensing against the pain, gently explore softening around it on the exhale, as if making more room in the surrounding tissue.

Alternate between:

Narrow focus right in the painful area.

Wide focus including neutral/pleasant areas (e.g., hands, face, places of contact with the bed or chair).

This helps decenter from "I am pain" to "Pain is present within a larger field of experience."

Relating differently to aversion

When aversion shows up ("I can't stand this"), guide noticing these as mental events: "This is a thought," "I have an urge, an emotions," "my body is tightening."

Briefly label them ("resistance," "fear," "anger") and return to sensing, not storytelling.

Closing the practice

After scanning your whole body, rest in a sense of your body as a whole, breathing.

End with a brief intentional phrase, e.g., "I notice this pain with as much kindness and patience as possible."

This MSBR practice helps people with chronic pain by teaching them ways to relate differently to their pain, reducing its psychological impact and emotional distress, and improving quality of life through structured mindfulness practices. It helps lessen the intensity and interference of pain by fostering mindful awareness instead of avoidance or excessive control. Avoidance of suffering generally causes more suffering because rather than dealing with the psychological impact of the pain, avoidance of it can mean that the underlying cause could worsen without your attention. MBSR participants learn to observe pain sensations in an accepting, nonjudgmental way, which decreases emotional suffering and the "struggle" against pain, which can be exhausting.

Genetics and Self-Hatred

The question has been raised as to the role of genetics in self-hatred. There is no direct evidence that self-hatred is inherited; however, there are some components that might be influenced by genes. For instance, studies consistently show that pain tolerance runs in families, with both pain sensitivity and chronic pain risk being influenced by many genes. Environmental and psychological factors also interact with genetics, contributing to the overall experience of pain.

Another factor that might be influenced by genetics is your temperament. Temperament is your natural predisposition or characteristic way of behaving, reacting emotionally, and approaching the world, elements that are often considered to be the biological foundation of your personality. It is an innate, inborn style of emotional responsiveness and behavioral patterns that is evident from infancy and forms the groundwork for the development of your personality throughout your life.

Practicing Self-Compassion

Practicing self-compassion in everyday life doesn't always require grand gestures—it's often the small, mindful moments that make the biggest difference. These small actions can improve your health and sense of well-being, making them a way to support your foundational needs, biologically, mentally, and emotionally. Here are some simple everyday actions that are forms of kindness to the self from morning to evening:

Morning

Gentle wake-up: Instead of jolting awake to a harsh alarm, try a softer tone or a gradual light alarm. Take a deep breath and set a kind intention for the day.

Hydrate first thing: Before rushing into tasks, drink a glass of water to nourish your body.

Eat mindfully: Pause for a moment before eating to acknowledge your meal, even if it's just a snack.

No food guilt: If you indulge, remind yourself that enjoyment is part of being human—no need for shame.

At Work/School

Take micro-breaks: Stand up, stretch, or close your eyes for 30 seconds between tasks.

Set realistic expectations: Instead of "I must finish everything," try "I'll do what I can today."

Celebrate small wins: Acknowledge even minor progress—sending an email, making a call, or just showing up. Each day this week, write down one moment—no matter how small—when you felt even a little bit of acceptance or kindness toward yourself.

Move

Stretch like a cat: Move in whatever way feels good—no pressure to "exercise perfectly."

Soothing touch: Rub your own shoulders, hold your own hand, or give yourself a gentle hug.

Comfortable clothes: Choose outfits that make you feel at ease, not just "presentable."

Socially

Say no gracefully: Decline an invite or request without over-explaining—your energy matters.

End draining conversations early: "I need to step away for a bit" is self-care.

Limit self-criticism after socializing: Instead of replaying awkward moments, remind yourself, "I was human today."

Evening

Unplug early: Give yourself screen-free time to transition to rest.

Kind self-reflection: Instead of "I didn't do enough," try "I survived today, and that's enough."

Cozy ritual: Sip tea, listen to calming music, or use a warm blanket to signal rest.

Activity 7.1: Burdensomeness and Belongingness (IPTS Model)

Of the components of the IPTS, the two key drivers of suicidal behavior as it pertains to self-hatred are perceived burdensomeness and failed belongingness. Use this worksheet to explore these themes in your life.

A. Perceived burdensomeness

- Do you feel that you are a burden to others?

  ____

  ____

  ____

  ____

- What are the thoughts and words that show up when you are feeling like a burden?

  ____

  ____

  ____

  ____

- Are there particular times and situations when the feeling of burdensomeness shows up?

  ____

  ____

  ____

  ____

- Are there particular people that elicit the feeling of burdensomeness (can include loved ones, therapists, work colleagues)?

____

- How does the burdensomeness impact your relationships with the people you just listed?

____

- How does the feeling of burdensomeness impact your mood, your behaviors?

____

B. Failed belongingness

- Do you feel isolated even when you are surrounded by people?

____

- Do you feel like you don't belong to any group, including your family?

____

- What specific events or experiences contributed to those feelings?

- How do you cope with loneliness, emptiness, or disconnection?

- How does feeling that you don't belong contribute to your self-hatred?

Activity 7.2: Physical and Emotional Pain and Chronic Illness

Answer the following questions to determine how chronic pain or illness plays a role in your self-image, thinking patterns, and emotions.

- Do you experience chronic physical pain, or do you have a chronic illness?

- How has it affected your self-image?

- Do you notice a relationship between emotional pain and your ability to tolerate physical pain?

- When you are in emotional pain, do you experience physical pain differently?

- What are the ways that you judge yourself and those around you?

- Have you experienced invalidation or even outright skepticism and dismissal from the medical system?

- How have such experiences impacted your self-evaluation and tied into self-hatred?

____

____

____

____

Activity 7.3: Genetics, Temperament, and Self-Hatred

As noted, while there is no direct evidence that self-hatred is inherited, some traits like pain tolerance or temperament can be influenced by genetics.

- Have you noticed patterns of emotional sensitivity or pain tolerance in your family?

____

____

____

____

- How might your temperament or biology play a role in your emotional life?

____

____

____

____

- And as a consequence, how has this impacted your sense of self and contributed to your self-hatred?

____

____

____

____

- Are there ways your biology has made coping with life's challenges harder?

Activity 7.4: Mindful Awareness of Pain and Self-Hatred

Practice noticing when physical or emotional pain triggers self-hating thoughts. Use mindfulness to observe these thoughts and sensations without judgment. Write down what you notice:

- What is the pain?

- What thoughts arise?

- How can you respond with validation and self-compassion instead of self-criticism?

Activity 7.5: Noticing Smaller Moments of Self-Compassion

Write down your own schedule to help you plan to have purposeful moments of self-compassion. To get the most of them, be sure to approach them with mindfulness instead of like a to-do list. Over time, these can become habits.

Day	**Moments of Self-Acceptance**		
	Morning	**Daytime**	**Evening**
Monday			
Tuesday			
Wednesday			
Thursday			
Friday			

(continued)

(continued)

Saturday

Sunday

Key Points

- While no direct genetic link to self-hatred exists, genetics may influence components like pain tolerance and temperament that contribute to vulnerability.
- The IPTS identifies key risk factors: perceived burdensomeness, thwarted belongingness, and acquired capability for suicide.
- Chronic physical and emotional pain can intensify self-hatred by limiting activities, fostering self-criticism, and reinforcing feelings of being a burden.
- Mindfulness-based stress reduction (MBSR) helps people relate differently to pain, reducing its psychological impact without avoiding it.
- Small daily acts of self-compassion (gentle wake-ups, mindful eating, realistic expectations, celebrating small wins) can gradually improve well-being.

Part 3

Self-Hatred in Mental Health

Self-hatred is linked to many mental health conditions, including borderline personality disorder, eating disorders, depression, anxiety, and others. If you have a mental health diagnosis, Chapters 8 and 9 will help you understand how it is connected to self-loathing. If you do not have a diagnosis, but still struggle with self-hatred, please read Chapter 10, which explores the relationship between self-hatred and certain personality traits, including narcissism, perfectionism, people pleasing, and bullying. The Part 3 Activity here will help prepare you for the work ahead.

Part 3 Activity: Self-Hatred and My Mental Health Diagnosis

Reflect on your mental health history and current challenges. Use the prompts below to explore how self-hatred might connect with your experiences.

1. What mental health diagnoses have you received (if any)?

____

____

____

____

2. In what ways does self-hatred show up alongside your symptoms or diagnoses?

3. Are there times when self-hatred feels stronger or weaker depending on your mood or diagnosis?

4. Do you notice differences between "episodic" self-hatred (e.g., during depression) and "core" self-hatred (persistent, regardless of mood)?

Chapter 8

Borderline Personality Disorder and Self-Hatred

Chapter Summary

This chapter may not apply to everyone. It's critically important that you don't self-diagnose. If what you read in Chapter 8 of *I Hate Myself* overlaps with your symptoms, the best thing to do is consult with a mental health professional who has experience with borderline personality disorder (BPD). The exercises in this chapter are designed for people to complete with a therapist, so skip this chapter if it doesn't feel relevant or if you feel uncertain about whether you have an undiagnosed mental health condition.

People with BPD often experience severe emotional pain. Although it is not listed as a symptom in the Diagnostic and Statistical Manual of Mental Disorders (DSM), chronic, severe self-hatred is considered a hallmark feature in BPD, often experienced as immutable and deeply ingrained. These feelings are closely associated with toxic shame, emotional dysregulation, self-harm, and suicide attempts.

While BPD criteria can appear in hundreds of combinations, there are five areas of functioning that BPD tends to impact: emotional regulation, relationships, impulsivity, cognitive distortions, and sense of self. To be diagnosed with BPD, a person must meet at least five of the following criteria:

1. Fear of abandonment, whether it is real or not.
2. Intense and unstable relationships that swing between idealizing someone and criticizing every aspect of them.
3. A sense of self that fluctuates, or having no solid sense of self at all.
4. Impulsive and potentially risky behaviors.
5. Suicidal and self-injurious behavior.
6. Frequent and intense mood episodes.

7. Frequent feelings of emptiness or disconnection.
8. Intense and excessive anger, which can lead to the destruction of property or physical fights.
9. Dissociation, the sense of not feeling real or that the rest of the world isn't real.

I Hate Myself and this workbook are not diagnostic tools, so if these criteria resonate with you, please speak with a qualified therapist. If you experience suicidal thoughts, please immediately contact someone you trust. Suicide is never the solution.

In the past, there were no dedicated treatments for BPD. While new treatments have a significant positive impact and reduce many people's symptoms, they often do not target self-hatred specifically. Including exercises that address self-hatred can have a meaningful impact on their well-being.

Key Definitions and Concepts

- **Borderline personality disorder (BPD):** A mental health disorder that affects how people regulate their emotions, perceive themselves and others, and control their behaviors leading to negative effects on life functioning.
- **Sense of self:** Someone's personal experience of their own identity as a distinct person. It includes their self-awareness, self-boundaries, and idea of agency. It should remain relatively consistent, even though personality traits, relationships, and environment can change over time.
- **Dissociation:** A person's feeling that they aren't real or that the rest of the world isn't real; a sense of being detached from reality.
- **Emotional dysregulation:** This is a person's inability to manage and control their emotions effectively and can include difficulties in understanding and labeling their own emotions and then regulating emotions that can feel disproportionate to the triggering event.

Many of the exercises in this book may seem repetitive, and they are because continuous erosion of self-hatred happens through continuous focus. Every moment is a new opportunity to tackle self-hatred in therapy because being present allows you to notice and interrupt habitual self-critical thoughts, choose a more compassionate response, and gradually reshape your self-narrative. Mindfulness and therapeutic interventions encourage responding to your negative self-talk in real time, rather than being trapped by your old patterns of thinking and self-perception. Ask yourself questions like, "Is this belief about myself even true right now, or is it something I've carried from the past?" This type of question opens space to challenge and reframe negative beliefs.

You'll notice that Chapters 8 and 9 are different because they don't contain warm-up activities or additional readings. Instead, they focus on helping you and your therapist prepare to begin discussing your self-hatred together. After you review this chapter, look at Chapter 10 and decide with your therapist which activities there are also relevant to your individual needs. Use these activities with your therapist to open up direct conversations about self-hatred, assess its impact, and collaboratively develop treatment plans.

Activity 8.1: Exploring Self-Hatred in BPD

BPD often involves intense, persistent self-hatred, which together with unstable relationships, an unstable sense of self, and frequent intense and painful mood swings, makes the risk of suicidal behavior and self-destructiveness higher than for many other conditions. If you have been diagnosed with BPD, reflect on the following experiences:

1. Do you relate to feeling a persistent sense of being "bad," "broken," or "unlovable"?

   ____

   ____

   ____

   ____

2. How does the fear of abandonment or unstable relationships impact your self-view?

   ____

   ____

   ____

   ____

3. Have you noticed impulsive or self-destructive behaviors linked to self-hatred?

4. After impulsive actions, typically behaviors that are consistent with your value system, do you notice emotions or thoughts tied to self-hatred?

5. If you are in therapy, does your therapy offer skills to deal with intense emotions, volatile relationships, and potentially self-harming behaviors?

Activity 8.2: Taking the First Step Toward Change

Identify one belief or behavior related to self-hatred that you're willing to question or challenge this week.

1. Commit to talking to your therapist about self-hatred. When will you do this, and what will you say?

2. What small act of self-kindness can you try, even if it feels uncomfortable?

3. Other than your therapist, who else can you ask for support as you begin this work?

Activity 8.3: Naming and Sharing Self-Hatred

If you've never discussed self-hatred in therapy, use this activity to prepare.

1. How would you describe your experience of self-hatred to a therapist?

2. What are your fears about bringing it up?

3. What do you hope might change if you talk about it openly?

Activity 8.4: Mindfulness and Self-Compassion Practice

Your therapist should work with you to normalize the difficulty of discussing self-hatred and validate your experience. Follow their guidance to integrate dialectical behavior therapy (DBT), acceptance and commitment therapy (ACT), cognitive behavior therapy (CBT), and mindfulness skills, as appropriate, focusing on acceptance and change.

To answer the following questions, notice how you talk to yourself about self-hatred:

1. What are specific words and phrases you use?

____

____

____

____

2. For each word or phrase, practice responding with a kind, supportive, or validating tone, as you would to a friend. Alternatively, what are less hurtful words that you could use?

____

____

____

____

3. Write down one self-compassionate statement you can use when self-hatred arises. Something like, "I was taught to hate myself, but I can be kind to myself today by doing XYZ."

____

____

____

____

Key Points

- Chronic, severe self-hatred is a hallmark feature of BPD, closely linked to toxic shame, emotional dysregulation, and self-harm.
- BPD diagnosis requires at least five symptoms, including fear of abandonment, unstable relationships, fluctuating sense of self, impulsivity, and intense mood episodes.
- Every moment in therapy offers opportunity to challenge self-hatred by noticing and interrupting habitual self-critical thoughts in real time.
- Naming and sharing self-hatred openly with a therapist is a crucial first step toward change, despite fears about discussing it.
- Self-compassion practice, even when uncomfortable, is essential for countering the harsh inner critic common in BPD.

Other Psychiatric Diagnoses and Self-Hatred

Chapter Summary

I'll repeat my note from Chapter 8: This chapter might not be for everyone, and it's important that people don't self-diagnose. If what you read in Chapter 9 of *I Hate Myself* resonates with you, please consult with a mental health professional who has experience the symptoms you recognize in yourself. The exercises in this chapter are designed for people to complete with a therapist, so skip this chapter if it doesn't feel relevant or if you feel uncertain about whether you have an undiagnosed mental health condition.

Key Definitions and Concepts

- **Eating disorder:** A mental health condition identified by persistent abnormal thoughts about food, eating, or body image that affects physical health and daily life. Eating disorders typically involve restricting food intake (anorexia), binge eating, and/or compensating for caloric intake through purging (bulimia) or excessive exercise.
- **Disordered eating:** Disordered eating describes a range of irregular eating behaviors that may or may not include the diagnosis of a specific eating disorder.
- **Body image:** A person's subjective beliefs and emotions about their body, and their perception of their physical appearance, shape, and size. It includes actions they take to examine, alter, or conceal their body.
- **Body dysmorphic disorder (BDD):** A mental health condition where someone becomes fixated on perceived flaws in their physical appearance that others are unlikely to notice.

- **Obsessive compulsive disorder (OCD):** A mental health disorder that causes recurring, intrusive, unwanted thoughts or images (obsessions) or urges to engage in repetitive behavior (compulsions).
- **Depression:** A mental health condition diagnosed by a change in functioning caused by five or more recognized symptoms, including at least one of the following: (1) depressed mood, (2) loss of interest or pleasure.
- **Anxiety:** Excessive fear or worry that something bad will happen. It interferes with daily life and can include physical symptoms like accelerated heart rate, psychomotor agitation, and others.

Self-hatred, and related negative self-evaluations like self-blame and self-criticism, is highly prevalent across several mental health conditions, but the exact rates and manifestations vary depending on the disorder. It often appears as persistent self-criticism, intense negative self-judgment, or feelings of worthlessness and shame, which can be core symptoms or strong risk factors in these diagnoses. For instance:

- **Eating disorders (EDs):** High levels of self-hatred, poor self-image, and self-blame are highly prevalent in most eating disorder diagnoses, including anorexia, bulimia, and binge eating disorder. Low self-esteem and self-hatred not only puts people at risk for developing eating disorders but also sustains them over time.
- **Body dysmorphic disorder (BDD):** Many patients with EDs also struggle with BDD, although not everyone with poor body image has a formal eating disorder, even if they engage in disordered eating. Many people who have a poor body image also have core self-hatred.
- **Obsessive compulsive disorder (OCD):** Many people with OCD experience intense self-criticism and self-blame linked to their intrusive thoughts and compulsive behaviors. This can be particularly true if the nature of the intrusive thoughts are taboo, such sacrilegious thoughts or thoughts of harming others, especially your children. People with OCD can internalize their intrusive symptoms as signs of personal defectiveness, which leads to deep feelings of shame, guilt, and self-hatred.

- **Depression:** Self-hatred is a common symptom of major depressive disorder (MDD), with most patients reporting frequent feelings of inadequacy, low self-worth, or intense self-blame. Studies show that self-blaming emotions, including self-disgust and shame, occur in over 80 percent of people with MDD, tightly linked with depressed mood and hopelessness.
- **Anxiety disorders:** Self-hatred can exacerbate anxiety symptoms and is frequently seen in people with social anxiety, often preceding or compounding anxious thoughts. People with anxiety may believe they are inherently unworthy, fueling a cycle of self-criticism and excessive worry about being judged or punished.
- **Other conditions:** Self-hatred is present in many personality and mood disorders, often linked to persistent negative self-image and guilt, which is common in body dysmorphic disorder (BDD) and some cases of post-traumatic stress disorder (PTSD), especially when the person feels that they are to blame for the trauma that happened to them.

Table 9.1 summarizes the key points of each of these disorders, including their prevalence, manifestation, and effects.

Table 9.1 Self-Hatred in Psychiatric Disorders

Condition	Self-Hatred Prevalence/ Manifestation	Notable Impacts
Depression (MDD)	80%+ experience persistent self-blame, inadequacy, low self-worth	Suicidal ideation, severe impairment
Anxiety disorders	Frequent, intensifies symptoms, especially social anxiety	Avoidance, isolation
BPD	Chronic, severe, often seen as a barrier to recovery	Emotional dysregulation, unstable relationships, self-harm and suicidal behaviors
Eating disorders	High; self-hate, blame, low self-love in most cases	Maintains illness, worsens outcomes

(continued)

Table 9.1 *(continued)*

Condition	Self-Hatred Prevalence/ Manifestation	Notable Impacts
OCD	Common: Flawed sense of self, shame and guilt	Compulsive behaviors to "prevent" the intrusive thoughts from become actions, isolation
Other mood/ personality diagnoses (see Chapter 10)	Common, especially with perceived defect disorders	Increased shame, linked to suicidality

Perhaps most importantly, self-hatred is commonly seen in people experiencing suicidal ideation, regardless of diagnosis, and should be a key question in any psychiatric evaluation of people with suicidal behaviors. If you have thoughts of suicide or self-harm, immediately contact someone you trust, call the Suicide and Crisis Lifeline (988) or go to your nearest emergency room. Suicide is never the answer.

One important last point to note: Although these are individual diagnoses, many people who struggle with mental illness can have with two or more of these diagnoses, making the burden of care all the more challenging. Having two or more diagnoses is also known as having comorbidities.

Eating Disorders and Body Dysmorphic Disorder

There is a significant link between eating disorders, body image, and self-hatred. Because a very common experience of people with eating disorders is dissatisfaction with body image, this dissatisfaction can intensify to the point of self-hatred. In fact, self-hatred and negative body image are deeply interconnected, with self-hatred often both arising from and fueling dissatisfaction and shame about your physical appearance. This can be aggravated by contemporary and societal views where negative body image can be linked to internalized standards of beauty and self-worth, at times created by external images and social media expressions, and then, when the internalized standards are unmet, they can provoke harsh self-criticism and contempt toward the self.

Obsessive Compulsive Disorder

People with OCD frequently believe that their intrusive thoughts or compulsions reveal who they truly are, fueling self-loathing. The pressure of trying to control or neutralize these disturbing thoughts often leads to frustration and self-judgment when effort feels futile. In this context, people may isolate themselves to hide their symptoms, intensifying feelings of loneliness and self-hate.

Depression

As mentioned earlier, studies show that more than 80 percent of depressed patients experience self-blaming emotions, including guilt, especially affective guilt, which is a general feeling of unworthiness, self-disgust, persistent feelings of inadequacy, or a pervasive sense of having done something wrong. These symptoms co-occur with core depressive symptoms like hopelessness and depressed mood. During a depressive episode, if self-hatred manifests with hopelessness, the risk of suicidal thoughts and behaviors is significant. Self-hatred in depression is often episodic and transient and often associated with the depressive episode, while core self-hatred tends to be more persistent. Of course, as mentioned earlier, people can have more than one condition.

Self-Kindness and Psychiatric Diagnoses

These are not all the psychiatric diagnoses where self-hatred is a common feature, and there are many people with self-hatred who do not have a psychiatric diagnosis. In this chapter and Activity 8.1, you will review a practice that can help irrespective of diagnosis, or if you have no diagnosis at all. The idea here is that even if core and enduring self-hatred is not present, all instances of negative self-evaluation should be addressed on a regular basis for two reasons: The first is in order to bring awareness to all negative self-evaluations and address them early, and the second is that all these practices are ones that are central to building a skill set against self-hatred.

For many people with core self-hatred, and even for those in the depths of a depressive episode, the idea of practicing self-compassion can seem daunting at best and impossible or even invalidating at worst—invalidating because people with core self-hatred fundamentally do not believe that they deserve compassion. You nevertheless need to practice if you want to overcome self-hatred.

Here are some ideas to show kindness to yourself when struggling with mental illness:

1. **1.** Practice self-talk that is kinder than the negative talk you are currently using: Gently remind yourself that suffering is part of being human and that you deserve care and understanding, not criticism, when things are hard. Repeat supportive phrases like: "I am doing my best," "It's okay to need help," or "I am worthy of kindness." Another way is to talk to yourself as you would to a friend going through a tough time.
2. **2.** Engage in a small act of self-care: Give yourself permission to rest, take a shower, eat something nourishing, or spend time in an environment that feels comforting or safe. Do a pleasurable or comforting activity—listen to music, take a walk, or spend time in nature. These acts are kind self-actions, and you deserve them.
3. **3.** Pause and breathe mindfully: Take a few slow, deep breaths, placing your hand over your heart or giving yourself a gentle hug, and acknowledge your feelings without judgment.

I Hate Myself and this workbook are not diagnostic tools, so if these criteria resonate with you, please speak with a qualified therapist. If you experience suicidal thoughts, please immediately contact someone you trust. Suicide is never the solution.

As mentioned previously, many of the exercises in this book are repetitive, and they are because continuous erosion of self-hatred happens through continuous focus. Every moment is a new opportunity to tackle self-hatred in therapy because being present allows you to notice and interrupt habitual self-critical thoughts, choose a more compassionate response, and gradually reshape your self-narrative. Mindfulness and therapeutic interventions encourage responding to your negative self-talk in real time, rather than being trapped by your old patterns of thinking and self-perception. Ask yourself questions like, "Is this belief about myself even true right now, or is it something I've carried from the past?" This type of question opens space to challenge and reframe negative beliefs.

Like Chapter 8, this chapter doesn't contain warm-up activities or additional readings. Instead, it focuses on helping you and your therapist prepare to begin discussing your self-hatred together. After you review this chapter, look at Chapter 10 and decide with your therapist which activities there are also relevant to your individual needs. Use these activities with your therapist to open up direct conversations about self-hatred, assess its impact, and collaboratively develop treatment plans.

A note for the therapist: Use these worksheets to help clients differentiate between types of self-hatred, recognize the impact of diagnosis on self-view, and build self-compassion. Weave in DBT, ACT, CBT, and mindfulness practices as needed. Clearly, you would need to be skilled in these therapies in order to use them. Encourage clients to discuss their reflections and insights in session, and tailor interventions to their unique experiences. In all circumstances, the focus on targeting self-hatred must persist. The therapist must recognize their own impulse to avoid bringing up self-hatred.

Activity 9.1: Taking the First Step Toward Change

Identify one belief or behavior related to self-hatred that you're willing to question or challenge this week.

1. Commit to talking to your therapist about self-hatred. When will you do this, and what will you say?

 ____

 ____

 ____

 ____

2. What small act of self-kindness can you try, even if it feels uncomfortable?

 ____

 ____

 ____

 ____

3. Other than your therapist, who else can you ask for support as you begin this work?

____

____

____

____

Activity 9.2: Eating Disorders, Body Image, and Self-Hatred

Your therapist should work with you to normalize the difficulty of discussing self-hatred and eating disorders, and body dysmorphic disorder (BDD) can intensify self-hatred, especially through negative body image and self-comparison.

- How does dissatisfaction with your body affect your self-esteem and self-worth?

  ____

  ____

  ____

  ____

- If these are negative, does poor self-worth ever intensify to self-hatred?

  ____

  ____

  ____

  ____

- Do you notice a cycle between self-hatred and disordered eating or body-checking behaviors?

  ____

  ____

  ____

  ____

- How do comparisons with others impact your self-view?

- What feelings come up when you receive compliments or positive feedback about your appearance?

Activity 9.3: Self-Blame and Self-Compassion (CBT/ACT)

Self-blame is a common driver of self-hatred in eating disorders. Use this worksheet to challenge self-blaming thoughts.

- Write down a recent self-blaming thought (e.g., "It's my fault I feel this way").

- What evidence supports this thought?

- What evidence contradicts it?

- What would you say to a friend who had this thought?

- Can you replace the thought with a self-validating thought? (e.g., "Feeling guilt or shame after eating doesn't mean I'm a bad person. This is a sign I need kindness and help—not self-blame.")

Activity 9.4: OCD and Negative Self-Beliefs

People with OCD may interpret intrusive thoughts as evidence of being "bad" or "immoral," which can lead to significant negative self-evaluation, a sense of being flawed, and at times, self-hatred.

- Do you experience repetitive unwanted, intrusive thoughts?

- How do you judge or interpret them?

- What are the emotions that show when the thoughts arise?

- Do you tend to isolate or hide for fear that others will know your thoughts?

- Are there other behaviors that you do to prevent yourself as being seen by others or yourself as a bad person deserving negative judgments?

- Do you equate having these thoughts with being a bad person?

Activity 9.5: Depression and Self-Hatred

Reflect on your experience:

- What are the thoughts and changes in your sense of self that you experience when you are depressed?

- When you feel depressed, do feelings of worthlessness, self-disgust, or self-loathing increase?

- Do these feelings lift when your mood improves, or do they persist?

- How do you experience self-hatred differently during depressive episodes versus other times?

- If you have more than one mental health diagnosis where self-hatred shows up, how is the self-hatred similar and how is it different?

____

____

____

____

Activity 9.6: Building Self-Compassion Across Diagnoses (DBT/ACT/Mindfulness)

- With the above examples in mind, list three ways you can show kindness to yourself, particularly when you are struggling with mental health symptoms.

1. ____
2. ____
3. ____

- Practice a brief self-compassion meditation: Place your hand on your heart, take a deep breath, and repeat: "May I be kind to myself in this moment; may I feel peace, because I deserve peace; may I feel loved." If you need additional reinforcement, write the words down here:

____

____

____

____

- Identify one small act of self-care you can do today, regardless of your diagnosis.

____

____

____

____

Key Points

- Self-hatred appears across multiple diagnoses.
- In eating disorders and body dysmorphic disorder, negative body image and societal beauty standards fuel intense self-criticism and contempt.
- People with OCD may believe intrusive thoughts reveal their true character, leading to self-loathing and isolation to hide symptoms.
- Depression involves episodic self-hatred that co-occurs with hopelessness, while core self-hatred tends to be more persistent across diagnoses.
- Practicing kind self-talk, small acts of self-care, and mindful breathing can help counter self-hatred.

Chapter 10

Other Personality Traits and Self-Hatred

Chapter Summary

While there isn't much research on self-hatred, Chapter 10 of *I Hate Myself* looks at published studies that examine clinical topics that are often raised along with self-hatred. As with Chapters 8 and 9, do not use this to self-diagnose. If something feels relevant to you, use it as a starting point for a discussion with your therapist. All readers can benefit from the activities at the end of this workbook chapter, including who don't believe they have these personality traits.

This chapter discusses narcissism, perfectionism, people pleasing, and bullying. People with vulnerable narcissism are likely to have self-hatred because they have a sense of inferiority. They exhibit narcissistic behaviors and thoughts because they seek reassurance from and hope to compensate for their feelings of inadequacy. Narcissists seek external praise. When they do not receive constant admiration, they can find it difficult to overcome their self-loathing.

People with perfectionism are so focused on doing things perfectly that they experience extreme anxiety, humiliation, shame, and disappointment when things aren't perfect. They worry that others will judge them negatively if they do not perform perfectly in everything at all times. They are also dissatisfied if they are unable to meet their own high standards. Sometimes, perfectionism prevents them from completing tasks. Perfectionism can also harm relationships because people with perfectionism fear that people will perceive them as being flawed and reject them. Any kind of criticism, feedback, or rejection is seen as intolerable. This can lead to self-invalidation and even self-hatred.

People pleasing reflects the desire for positive attention (as seen in vulnerable narcissists) and reassurance (as seen in perfectionism). People pleasers tend to be extremely sensitive and observant of others, perceiving anything negative as dissatisfaction or criticism that they should fix by changing their behavior. Often, people pleasers learn their behavior from facing impossible standards or unrealistic expectations in childhood. This reliance on external validation can lead to self-hatred.

People who engage in bullying behavior were often exposed to violence in the home as children. In one study, 34% of children exposed to violence at home engaged in bullying, and almost all of the bullies (97%) said they were also victims of bullying. People who accept that they deserved the abuse are more likely to develop self-hatred. They may also conclude that it is acceptable to harm others. While self-hatred and bullying behavior is more prevalent in people who were abused as children, self-hatred alone does not correlate with bullying behavior.

Key Definitions and Concepts

- **Narcissism:** An unreasonably high sense of self-importance, a desire to be at the center of attention, and a desire for the admiration of others. People with narcissistic personality disorder often seem to love themselves to the exclusion of others and put themselves above everyone else. There are two types of narcissism:
  - **Grandiose narcissism:** Also known as overt narcissism; a subtype of narcissistic personality disorder characterized by a highly inflated sense of self-importance, entitlement, arrogance, and a persistent need for admiration. People with grandiose narcissism typically appear confident, assertive, and sometimes charismatic, but are also manipulative, dismissive of others, and lack genuine empathy.
  - **Vulnerable narcissism:** Also known as covert narcissism; a subtype of narcissistic personality characterized by a combination of narcissistic traits (such as self-centeredness and a need for admiration) with deep insecurity, low self-esteem, and hypersensitivity to criticism or rejection. While grandiose narcissists display obvious arrogance and entitlement, vulnerable narcissists present as introverted, self-conscious, anxious, and emotionally fragile.
- **Perfectionism:** A person's inability to be satisfied with their daily activities and performance of tasks because the person perceives them as imperfect.

Like Chapter 8, this chapter doesn't contain warmup activities or additional readings. Instead, it focuses on

Connecting with Your Future Self

An exercise that has worked for those with lived experience of self-hatred and related personality traits, including narcissism and perfectionism, is that of connecting with their future self. Meeting your future self can guide you toward acceptance in the present by offering perspective, hope, and actionable wisdom, a wisdom that reframes how you relate to yourself now. Here's how this process works:

1. **Inspiration and encouragement:** Your future self, the person that you want to be a week, a month or a year from now, does not want to be hating themselves. Visualizing and even talking to your future self, one who no longer hates themselves and instead has compassion for you today, helps you receive inspiration and encouragement for the challenges you face today. By imagining a wiser, more compassionate version of yourself, you can access guidance and reassurance that self-acceptance is possible—even if it feels distant right now.
2. **Clarity on what truly matters:** Connecting with your future self allows you to clarify your core values and long-term goals. This perspective helps you see beyond your current struggles or self-judgments, focusing instead on the bigger picture of who you want to become. When you know what your future self values, it becomes easier to accept your present self as a work in progress, rather than a finished product. Your future self does not value self-hatred. Be honest with yourself, is self-hatred truly a value of yours today?
3. **Positive impact on present choices:** Imagine your future self writes you a letter. Can you write that letter? Research shows that building a relationship with your future self can positively influence your current decisions, making it easier to choose self-kindness and acceptance over self-criticism. When you see yourself as someone who is growing and evolving toward that person in the future, you're more likely to treat yourself with patience and compassion in the present.
4. **Encouragement to take small, accepting steps:** Imagining your future self doesn't require envisioning a perfect, completely self-loving distant version of you. Even picturing yourself being a little bit kinder, a little less harsh on yourself, a few months from now can help you identify small,

manageable steps you can take now to move toward acceptance. This approach emphasizes progress over perfection and helps you accept where you are today as a valid part of your journey.

5. **Embodying self-acceptance:** Imagine that you could be in the mind of your future self and that you could know how they think, feel, and act. Imagine that person being kinder to you the way that you would be kinder to the child who was hurt. You can practice embodying qualities like self-acceptance and self-compassion right now. This experiential exercise helps you feel what it's like to accept yourself, making it easier to bring up those feelings more regularly into your daily life, and particularly when self-hatred is strong.

Nothing in the universe remains fixed. In dialectical behavior therapy (DBT), the concept of impermanence refers to the understanding that all emotions, thoughts, and experiences are temporary—they change and fade with time. This is no different from the concept of constant change in the field of physics which refers to the idea that the universe and all its physical phenomena are continuously evolving. Within every experience, there are changes and fluctuations. If you think of a body of water, the surface is never completely flat; sometimes there are tiny ripples, and at other times huge waves, but the water is never static. Similarly, it can feel as if self-hatred is constant, but it isn't. There will be times when you feel it more intensely and other times, when it is less obvious, even if it is there all the time. For some people with lived experience, noticing these shifts can help.

Pros and Cons: A DBT Approach

Another tool that people with lived experience have found helpful is the pros and cons skill of DBT. The goal is to empower you to methodically and realistically assess the advantages and disadvantages of making a choice. DBT applies a four-way grid system, allowing for a clear and comprehensive evaluation of the options at hand (Figure 10.1). This approach helps you weigh your choices against your long-term goals and values, and increase the likelihood that your decision is aligned with the life that you want to build. For example, say you were deciding on whether to work on self-hatred or not. There are four evaluations to complete. In this example, there is only one item listed per pro and con; however Activity 10.9 contains a blank worksheet where you should list all the pros and all the cons in each box of the grid.

1. Pros of working on self-hatred: A pro might be that exploring self-hatred allows you to understand and challenge the deep-rooted negative beliefs about yourself as an essential step for healing and growth.	**2. Cons of working on self-hatred:** You might feel that addressing self-hatred is too emotionally painful and that it will provoke strong anxiety or vulnerability, leading to setbacks in therapy, and feel that it is a waste of time as you feel that it is not something that can change.
3. Pros of not addressing self-hatred: By choosing to not address self-hatred you don't have to dive into painful memories which could retraumatize or increase distress.	**4. Cons of not addressing self-hatred:** You won't develop the tools to build self-compassion and reduce harsh self-criticism, and you won't learn how to treat yourself with kindness and validation.

Figure 10.1 The four-way grid.

A note for the therapist: Use these worksheets to help clients differentiate between types of self-hatred, recognize the impact of diagnosis on self-view, and build self-compassion. Weave in DBT, ACT, CBT, and mindfulness practices as needed. Clearly, you would need to be skilled in these therapies in order to use them. Encourage clients to discuss their reflections and insights in session, and tailor interventions to their unique experiences. In all circumstances, the focus on targeting self-hatred must persist. The therapist must recognize their own impulse to avoid bringing up self-hatred.

Activity 10.1: Self-Blame and Self-Compassion (CBT/ACT)

Self-blame is a common driver of self-hatred in eating disorders. Use this worksheet to challenge self-blaming thoughts.

- Write down a recent self-blaming thought (e.g., "It's my fault I feel this way").

____

____

____

____

- What evidence supports this thought?

____

____

____

____

- What evidence contradicts it?

____

____

____

____

- What would you say to a friend who had this thought?

____

____

____

____

- Can you replace the thought with a self-validating thought? (e.g., "Feeling guilt or shame after eating doesn't mean I'm a bad person. This is a sign I need kindness and help—not self-blame.")

____

____

____

____

Activity 10.2: Building Self-Compassion Across Diagnoses (DBT/ACT/Mindfulness)

- With the above examples in mind, list three ways you can show kindness to yourself, particularly when you are struggling with mental health symptoms.

1. ______________________________
2. ______________________________
3. ______________________________

- Practice a brief self-compassion meditation: Place your hand on your heart, take a deep breath, and repeat: "May I be kind to myself in this moment; may I feel peace, because I deserve peace; may I feel loved." If you need additional reinforcement, write the words down here:

____

____

____

____

- Identify one small act of self-care you can do today, regardless of your diagnosis.

____

____

____

____

Activity 10.3: Noticing Shifts in Self-Hatred

- List situations when your self-hatred is strongest (e.g., after criticism, when you are alone, when you are comparing yourself to others).

____

____

____

____

- List times when self-hatred is less intense (e.g., doing something you enjoy, helping others, being creative).

____

____

____

____

- Similarly, list the people in your life or in your memory who intensify the feeling of self-hatred.

____

____

____

____

- List the ones who life you up and who make you feel better about yourself.

____

____

____

____

- Are there activities or situations that help reduce your self-hatred, even if briefly?

____

____

____

____

- Do you have any choice in how you spend your time and or with the people you choose to be.

____

____

____

____

- Do you choose situations that are more likely to lead to self-hatred because you do not believe that you deserve any better?

____

____

____

____

- Can you commit to spend a little more time with people who care about you and doing the things that make you feel better about yourself and less time with the people who hurt you and doing the things that make you feel worse about yourself?

____

____

____

____

Activity 10.4: Comparing Yourself to "Bad People"

For some with lived experience, another helpful exercise is comparing themselves to historical figures who have committed truly terrible acts. Many people with core self-hatred can believe that they are the worst person ever and feel as if the world would be better off had they never been born. Because they are so consumed by their self-hatred, they cannot see their innate worth, and nor can they see that they are not even anywhere close to how awful other human beings have been in the past or even are, in the present.

- List people you consider truly evil (historical figures, criminals, etc.).

____

____

____

____

- Write down what makes them evil in your view.

- What are the actions you have done that make you evil or bad?

- Compare your actions and intentions to those of the truly evil, in terms of mass destruction, theft of property, gross and intentional disregard for the lives of others.

- Does this reframe your view of yourself?

- Are you as truly terrible as you are believing yourself to be?

- In the pantheon of really evil people, do you even come close?

- List a few qualities that make you different from the truly bad people in the world.

Coming out of this dark exercise, there is the flipside, and that is the task of seeing the qualities in yourself that you see in the people that you admire. See Activity 10.5.

Activity 10.5: Identifying and Owning Positive Qualities

- List the names of people in your life that you admire, whether past or present, and list the qualities you admire in them.

- Do you possess any of these qualities?

- How do these qualities show up in your life, even in small ways?

- Can you allow yourself to admire these parts of yourself as you admire them in other people?

- Can you fully hate yourself for having those admirable qualities, when you don't have any hatred for the people that you hold in high regard?

Activity 10.6: Dismissing Past Bullies and Tormentors

In this exercise, the recognition that some with lived experience have, that part of what keeps self-hatred alive is the seeming permanence that past bullies and tormentors live in their minds. Letting go of them is not easy, and it is much harder if they continue to exist in your present life. The work involves facing and processing painful memories, reframing harmful beliefs, and recognizing that many of them are no longer a part of your life today. Carrying them with you from the past into the present moment is also carrying the weight of all their hurt into today. Do they deserve to occupy so much space in your mind?

Answer the following questions to help yourself dismiss past tormentors.

- Who is a person or group of people whose criticism or bullying still echoes in your mind?

____

____

____

____

- What were the things that they said and did to you? If these actions led to significant trauma, you may need to process these in a trauma-focused therapy.

____

____

____

____

- If you saw them bullying a child similar to the way in which you were bullied and tormented, what would you say to them today if you could?

____

____

____

____

- How would you intervene?

____

____

____

____

- Are there people who could have intervened but who didn't? Do you blame them?

____

____

____

____

- Write a statement kicking them out of your mental space (e.g., "You don't get to live in my head anymore").

____

____

____

____

- Imagine them as spoiled food that you need to discard.

____

____

____

____

- This last part of this exercise may be very difficult, and is not necessary, but see if you can generate any compassion for your bullies and tormentors. Try to recognize that they, too, were caused by their circumstances and may have been bullied and tormented themselves, while recognizing that their actions toward you and others were still hurtful.

____

____

____

____

Activity 10.7: Realizing Self-Hatred Was Learned

One of the ideas that appears to resonate with many people who have lived experience is that they were not born hating themselves, but rather that the idea or feeling was learned. It changes the idea that you are fundamentally flawed and that self-hatred is a part of your DNA, but rather that ignorant and hurtful people convinced you that you were broken, even if they didn't recognize the ways in which their actions hurt you. Their actions may not have been intentional, but they caused damage nonetheless.

Answer the following questions to remind yourself that you learned your self-hatred. It is not an intrinsic part of you.

- Who were the people who taught you to hate yourself?

____

____

____

____

- What were their actions, inactions, statements, or non-verbal communications that led you to believe that you were not worth it?

____

____

____

____

- Did the constancy of the messaging teach you, and subsequently lead you to believe that you were, in fact, flawed and that the flaw was an unchangeable part of who you are as a person?

____

____

____

____

- What would you say to a child you cared about who received those same messages or experienced the same behaviors?

____

____

____

____

- Was there anyone in your life who did protect you?

____

____

____

____

- Can you challenge the belief that self-hatred is an unchangeable truth, and rather recognize that it was a lesson taught by ignorant and hurtful people?

____

____

____

____

Activity 10.8: Striving for Independence and Agency

Another idea that has worked for those with lived experience is that working for independence and self-advocacy can help reduce self-hatred because it helps you recognize your own authentic capabilities, to set and achieve personal goals, and to develop a self-confidence that isn't dependent on external approval, and this is how such striving can help:

- **It boosts your self-confidence:** Each independent decision, achievement, or problem you solve reinforces your belief in your personal ability, which enhances self-confidence and self-worth.
- **It promotes self-validation:** Relying less on others for approval means that you can feel your successes as your own, and then even if you don't fully succeed, you can validate that despite everything, you tried.
- **It encourages the pursuit of personal goals:** By focusing on a more independent life, you start the process of setting and attaining meaningful, self-chosen objectives, which are vital for feeling more capable and worthy.

Answer the following questions to help you get started:

- Make an honest appraisal of your strengths. For many people with self-hatred, they may be tempted to answer that they have none, and yet there are always qualities. You might be a loyal friend, or sibling. You might be a caring pet owner. You might be good at gardening or cooking. Maybe you are talented in art, music, or a sport.

- Recall a time you achieved something through your own effort.

- How did that accomplishment make you feel?

- What's one small goal you can strive for this week to build your sense of agency?

- Try to achieve even a part of the goal and follow that up with self-recognition, particularly if the goal is typically something that you find difficult to do.

- Step outside comfort zones, take risks, accept your successes as yours, and learn from your mistakes when need be. Do this as a way of expanding your trust in yourself. It is key not to judge yourself or be self-critical when things don't work out the way you want them to.

- Seek support when needed, but try to do so only after you have tried to solve a problem yourself, thereby increasingly taking responsibility for learning and decision-making.

Activity 10.9: Pros and Cons

Complete the following grid with all the pros and cons for you.

1. Pros of working on self-hatred:	2. Cons of working on self-hatred:

3. Pros of not addressing self-hatred:

4. Cons of not addressing self-hatred:

Key Points

- Vulnerable narcissism stems from deep insecurity and inferiority, with narcissistic behaviors used to seek reassurance and compensate for self-loathing.
- Perfectionism drives extreme anxiety about meeting impossibly high standards, with any criticism or perceived flaw triggering shame and self-invalidation.
- People pleasing reflects a desperate need for external validation, often learned from childhood experiences of impossible standards or unrealistic expectations.
- Connecting with a compassionate future self provides inspiration, clarity on values, and motivation to take small steps toward self-acceptance today.

Part 4

Treatment and Overcoming Barriers to Treatment

While there is little formal research on self-hatred, there is evidence that many treatment approaches can help people with self-loathing. This part helps you identify potential barriers to progress, and it offers a look at the therapist's perspective on treating self-hatred. It's important to remember that you are not alone. Not only do you have people in your life who are prepared to support you, but there are many other people who experience self-hatred. *I Hate Myself* includes their advice, and this workbook builds on that by giving you activities to practice the strategies that work best for you. Self-hatred can be hard to tackle, but with practice and support from your therapist, you can make progress in overcoming it and regaining control over your thoughts and life.

Part 4 Activity: Avatar of Confidence

Design a character who embodies your strengths. It can be a superhero, fantasy character, or simply a regular person who has all of your best qualities. Describe them here or if you have artistic ability, draw a picture of them highlighting your strengths.

When you feel small or lack confidence, channel your avatar to remind you of all your positive qualities to restore your sense of well-being.

Chapter 11

Targeting Self-Hatred

Chapter Summary

Addressing self-hatred is different from many other mental health experiences because there aren't any established, evidence-based therapies for self-hatred. However, based on my training and experience, the exercises I recommend in *I Hate Myself* and this companion workbook have the potential to reduce self-hatred, especially among people working with a qualified therapist.

Like many core beliefs, self-hatred emerges from our experiences in every aspect of life. It can be considered a harmful core belief, which causes significant stress and can be damaging to a person's well-being. There is a theory that core beliefs can even play a major role in depression and anxiety. Self-hatred can be especially challenging when the people who experience it do not consider it to be a core belief. For some, they see it as something unchangeable, an intrinsic part of who they are.

The way therapies are applied is important. If possible, people with self-loathing should work with a therapist who recognizes that self-hatred can be a distinct condition and a symptom of a disorder. Unless you and your therapist consider self-loathing as its own entity, it can be difficult to benefit from the activities and exercises in these books. It could even make someone feel like they failed at their treatment, which can make their self-hatred worse. Psychodynamic and relationally based therapies explore the role of early childhood experiences that likely created cognitive distortions and negative self-image, but this can also leave people with self-hatred feeling helpless to change their past. Behavioral therapies, on the other hand, can feel invalidating because it can appear as if all that is needed is for behavior to change, and behavioral change is very difficult in self-hatred.

Ultimately, only you have the power to overcome your self-hatred. The following approaches work best:

- Self-compassion and compassion-focused therapies (CFTs) to practice self-love as a way to improve well-being and reduce self-hatred.
- Acceptance and commitment therapy (ACT) tackles self-hatred by teaching you how to accept painful self-critical thoughts rather than trying to suppress or eliminate them, and then commit to actions that align with your personal values to build a richer, more meaningful life. ACT helps you defuse from harsh self-judgments, develop mindfulness, clarify values, and practice self-compassion.
- Mindfulness-based cognitive therapy (MBCT) addresses self-hatred by helping you develop a mindful, nonjudgmental awareness of your negative self-talk, teaching you to observe these thoughts as transient mental events rather than facts, and then to cultivate self-compassion to counter entrenched patterns of self-criticism.
- Cognitive behavior therapy (CBT) encourages people with self-hatred to acknowledge unhelpful or erroneous ways of thinking, identify learned patterns of unhelpful behavior, and learn more skilled and beneficial ways of coping. Dialect ic al behavior therapy (DBT) addresses self-hatred by blending acceptance and change strategies, with a particular focus on cultivating self-compassion, validating emotions, and targeting cycles of shame and self-invalidation.
- Mentalization-based therapy (MBT) addresses self-hatred by strengthening your capacity to understand and reflect upon your own mental states and those of others, breaking cycles of self-criticism and shame by fostering curiosity and empathy toward yourself.
- Schema therapy tackles self-hatred primarily through addressing maladaptive early schemas—a schema is a deep, enduring, and pervasive pattern of thought and feeling about yourself and the world that originates in childhood and is often maladaptive—especially the defectiveness/shame schema, which involves deep-seated beliefs that you are fundamentally flawed, unworthy, or defective. The therapy works by helping you identify these

negative core beliefs formed in childhood, understand the impact they have your on emotions and behaviors, and then gradually shift these schemas toward healthier, more compassionate views of self.

Key Definitions and Concepts

- **Acceptance-focused strategy:** Validating, compassionate therapy approaches that deeply recognize the suffering of the person. Although patients often feel very understood in these types of therapies, they can often be left wondering what action steps to take to overcome their self-hatred.
- **Change-focused strategy:** Therapy approaches that point out the flaw in the person's thinking and behavior and recommend ways to do things differently. Although these types of therapies can give you some very useful skills, they can also feel as if the therapy is suggesting that it is easy to overcome self-hatred.
- **Self-compassion:** Treating yourself with the kindness and understanding that you'd give a close friend who is struggling.
- **Self-contempt:** Feelings of hostility, contempt, disgust, or loathing that a person feels about themselves and leads to a rejection of the self as a person.
- **Decentering:** The ability to stand back and view a thought as a cognitive event rather than a fact.
- **Reattribution:** The practice of identifying the factors that have contributed to a negative outcome in a balanced way. It is used to change how you assign cause to negative events, shifting your focus from self-blame to a more balanced view that includes external factors.
- **Cognitive restructuring using thought records:** Reevaluating what you think about a specific situation in a practical way. This typically involves writing down your automatic thoughts about the situation, then considering the evidence to decide if your automatic thoughts are true.
- **Toxic shame:** A thought pattern of internalized shame that can impact schemas and core beliefs.

Ultimately, effective therapies all recognize that self-hatred has roots in childhood and is learned through repeated interactions that teach a child they are flawed. The key to overcoming negative core beliefs is to challenge them, and ultimately expose them as being untrue. The key is understanding that you have the power to change your ingrained thought patterns, which can create a positive feedback loop. Your therapist can help you find what approach works best for you.

Chapter 11 Warmup Activity: Notice Your Self-Talk

Notice how you talk to yourself about self-hatred and answer the following questions:

1. What are specific words and phrases you use?

    ____

    ____

    ____

    ____

2. For each word or phrase, practice responding with a kind, supportive, or validating tone, as you would to a friend. Alternatively, what are less hurtful words that you could use?

    ____

    ____

    ____

    ____

3. Write down one self-compassionate statement you can use when self-hatred arises—something like, "I was taught to hate myself but I can be kind to myself today by doing XYZ."

    ____

    ____

    ____

    ____

Radical Acceptance

One of the most powerful skills from DBT, which although powerful can be hard to practice, is that of *radical acceptance*. It is the practice of fully and completely accepting reality as it is—without judgment, resistance, or attempts to change it. It means acknowledging difficult situations, emotions, or experiences with your mind, body, and spirit, even when they are painful or uncomfortable.

Important things to note about radical acceptance:

- **It does not mean approval or liking the situation.** You don't have to agree with or support what's happening; you simply recognize the facts and stop fighting against reality. A steak is a steak whether you are a vegetarian or a carnivore. One can hate it, the other can love it, but it does not change the fact that the steak is a steak.
- **It is not resignation or giving up.** Instead of wasting energy on resisting what you can't change, radical acceptance allows you to focus on what you can control and act more effectively.
- **It involves letting go of emotional struggle.** By accepting what is, you reduce additional suffering caused by denial, anger, or frustration.
- **It allows full experience of emotions.** Acceptance means allowing yourself to feel pain, sadness, or anger without getting stuck in them or worsening your suffering by resistance.

Radical acceptance helps reduce emotional suffering by cutting through the resistance that amplifies pain, clarifying your focus, improving emotional regulation, and building resilience over time. Radical acceptance can be a powerful antidote to self-hatred by helping you end the inner battle against yourself and fostering deep self-compassion. Here's how it works:

- **Ends the internal war:** Radical acceptance means fully acknowledging your thoughts, feelings, flaws, and past experiences without judgment or denial—even the ones you dislike. Instead of criticizing yourself for your struggles or wishing you were different, you stop fighting reality, which quiets the inner critic and reduces emotional turmoil.

- **Normalizes imperfection:** By embracing all parts of yourself, you recognize that having flaws, painful emotions, or making mistakes is part of being human—not a personal failure. This mindset can seriously diminish the shame and harsh self-criticism at the root of self-hatred. Also, try to be consistent. Recognize that many times, the way you treat yourself for any perceived or real imperfections is NEVER the way you would treat others.
- **Fosters self-compassion:** Radical acceptance asks you to respond to your suffering with kindness, compassion, and patience—the same way you'd treat a friend, or a younger you, in pain. As you practice acceptance, you build the foundation for genuine self-care and emotional healing.
- **Shifts energy toward growth:** When you let go of self-judgment, you free up the mental and emotional energy once used to attack yourself. This energy can now be directed toward positive change and living more authentically.
- **Reduces suffering:** Anyone reading this book wants to suffer less. Acceptance does not mean approval but rather a willingness to see reality as it is. This reduces the distress and resistance that fuel self-hatred—and helps you move forward with greater peace, resilience, and clarity.

By practicing radical acceptance, you gradually transform self-hatred into self-understanding and self-compassion, allowing lasting change to emerge not from shame, but from a place of genuine care for yourself.

Especially if a traumatic past has caused your self-hatred, radical acceptance involves fully acknowledging reality—including the recollection of painful experiences and emotions—without judging them or trying to avoid them. Radical acceptance helps reduce the additional suffering that comes not from the trauma itself, but from struggling against its reality. You already experienced the trauma; playing it over and over in your mind only adds to suffering. You have been traumatized once, so no need to replay it. This is easier said than done; however, you can remind yourself that the trauma happened many years ago and that in this present moment it is not happening, and that you can accept that. The truth is that denying or fighting painful truths often deepens your suffering, and if you tend to blame yourself, this can worsen self-hatred. Acceptance allows emotional energy to be redirected toward healing and self-compassion.

To practice radical acceptance in DBT, you first notice and acknowledge your resistance to reality, then remind yourself that reality cannot be changed and that it is caused by whatever caused it. Further, that all causes have causes. Next, use your whole self—mind, body, and spirit—to accept the situation. You then practice behaviors associated with acceptance, engage in a thought experiment where you accept the unacceptable, notice body sensations, and allow difficult emotions to arise. Finally, remember that life is still worth living, even if what happened in your past happened. Here are the concrete steps:

1. **Observe your resistance to reality.** Catch yourself fighting or questioning reality, notice when you are thinking, "This shouldn't be this way" or "Why me?"
2. **Acknowledge reality's immutability and causes.** Remind yourself that you cannot change reality by rejecting it. Understand that no matter how unpleasant the situation, fighting it won't change the facts. Recognize its causes: Acknowledge that the present reality has a history and a cause that led to this present moment, which had to happen this way because of the causes.
3. **Practice acceptance with your whole self.** Use your mind, body, and spirit; employ strategies like accepting self-talk, smiling, mindfulness of your breath, and willing hands with unclenched hands and palms up.
4. **Engage in the DBT skill of opposite action.** Act as if you've accepted it. The way to do this is to list the behaviors you would engage in if you had accepted the facts, then do those behaviors as if you already have. If it is too hard to do, start with this seemingly silly exercise. Take an egg and drop it on your kitchen floor. The egg will break. This happened. Now you may judge the exercise and regret having broken an egg, but this does not change the reality that it is. The egg is broken. Write down your experience of rejecting what happened versus your feelings if you do accept reality.
5. **Practice a thought experiment.** Imagine believing the unbelievable: Rehearse in your mind what you would do if you accepted what seems unacceptable.

6. **Attend to your body sensations.** Stay grounded: Notice any sensations in your body—tension, aches, and pains—as you think about what you need to accept.
7. **Allow for difficult emotions to exist.** Don't suppress your feelings: Let feelings like sadness, disappointment, or grief arise without fighting them or suppressing them. Because everything changes, these will pass in time, and ironically, will persist if you fight them.
8. **Acknowledge life's worth.** Recognize that life can still be worth living, even in the presence of pain.

The following activities will get you started with radical acceptance and self-compassion. Starting with Activity 11.4, this chapter also includes group activities that have been adapted for individual therapy, but also lend themselves well to groups.

Activity 11.1: Radical Acceptance of the Present Moment

Identify something about yourself, something that happened to you, or something in your life that is hard to accept. Write it down here:

- Practice saying, "I accept that this is true right now, even if I don't like it." If it helps, write down that you accept this.

  ____

  ____

  ____

  ____

- What changes when you focus on accepting this moment, rather than fighting the past or fearing the future?

  ____

  ____

  ____

  ____

Activity 11.2: Practicing Core Self-Compassion

This exercise may seem obvious as a practice in overcoming self-hatred; however, for many people with core self-hatred, the very idea of practicing self-compassion seems impossible and invalidating. Nevertheless, ultimately you will get to the point where you can practice self-compassion and will welcome it. And so this exercise is included here as it comes from the practice of those with lived experience.

- List a daily act of self-care (e.g., eating, showering, resting).

____

____

____

____

- Reflect: Can you view this act as an expression of self-respect and compassion?

____

____

____

____

- Use kind language such as, "I am doing my best in this moment" or "This is a moment of suffering."

____

____

____

____

- Challenge harsh self-criticism by reminding yourself you did the best you could at the time when you were much younger and did not have support.

____

____

____

____

- Write a compassionate message to your younger self and to your present self.

Activity 11.3: Rewriting Your Story (Storytelling Exercise)

Next, it is important to note that not everyone feels that verbal or talking therapy is what works best for them. Some people like to express themselves through music, art, or writing. In this exercise, the task is to review past events through a different, and even a positive lens. This is a process called positive reframing. It does not invalidate what happened, but reframing can, for example, allow you to find meaning in traumatic experiences, and this in turn can help to promote optimism and help you develop a renewed sense of purpose and hope for the future. It supports your viewing challenges as learning opportunities, which, over time, motivates continued personal development.

- Write about a painful event from your past as you usually tell it ("the wrong side of storytelling").

- Now, rewrite the story with a focus on your resilience, growth, or compassion ("the right side of storytelling").

- How does this new narrative feel?

- If you are noticing self-invalidation, remember that you are not changing or denying what actually happened to you. You are considering whether, by only seeing the event through all the negative consequences, you might be missing a chance to see if something positive for your own personal growth might come out of it.

Activity 11.4: The Critic's Origin Story

In a therapy group, this activity would take place in the first session, which would focus on building safety and understanding self-hatred. In group therapy, participants would answer the question, then discuss their answers, following up in the next session. Individuals can also complete these activities and discuss their answers in one-on-one sessions.

- Question: When did you first feel not good enough? Whose voice does your inner critic mimic?

- Homework: Track self-critical thoughts in a journal.

Activity 11.5: The Courtroom

This is designed to be used in the second session of a therapy group. This session focuses on challenging cognitive distortions. In group therapy, participants would answer the question, then discuss their answers, following up in the next session. Individuals can also complete these activities and discuss their answers in one-on-one sessions.

- Question: Put your self-hatred on trial: What's the evidence for/against the belief "I'm worthless"?

- Homework: Replace one self-attack with a neutral statement (e.g., "I made a mistake" rather than "I'm stupid").

Activity 11.6: How Would You Treat a Friend?

This activity is designed to be used in the third session of a therapy group focused on self-hatred. The activity and session encourage clients to practice self-compassion. In group therapy, participants would answer the question, then discuss their answers, following up in the next session. Individuals can also complete these activities and discuss their answers in one-on-one sessions. In both cases, clients would write about a struggle as though they were advising a loved one.

1. Group Therapy Question: How would you treat another group member with core self-hatred?

   Individual Therapy Question: How would you treat a friend who expressed feelings of self-hatred?

   ____

   ____

   ____

   ____

2. Write about a struggle of your own as if you were advising a loved one.

   Compare your answers to questions 1 and 2 to your own self-talk.

   ____

   ____

   ____

   ____

   Homework: Perform one self-compassionate act (e.g., rest when tired).

   ____

   ____

   ____

   ____

Key Points

- Effective treatment requires recognizing self-hatred as both a distinct condition and a symptom, directly targeting it rather than hoping it resolves indirectly.
- Radical acceptance involves fully acknowledging reality without judgment or resistance, reducing suffering by ending the internal war against yourself.
- Self-compassion means treating yourself with the kindness you'd offer a close friend, not harsh criticism or conditional worth based on achievements.
- Small acts like rewriting your story with a resilience focus or writing a compassionate letter to your younger self can gradually shift self-narratives.

Chapter 12

Why Is Self-Hatred So Hard to Tackle?

Chapter Summary

As therapeutic approaches have advanced, many people facing debilitating mental health conditions have been helped by evidence-based approaches, but options for self-hatred have lagged. And yet while it may be difficult to find approaches to overcome self-hatred, it is absolutely possible. One way you and your therapist can make progress is by addressing possible barriers. One key barrier is that many therapists do not ask about self-hatred as part of the typical intake interview. If your therapist hasn't already asked about self-hatred, tell them about it. Explain it the same way you would any other symptom or concern.

Other barriers to addressing self-hatred can come from your own thought patterns and behaviors. Avoidance, comparison, and the certainty that nothing will change are three of the barriers people with self-hatred face. There are many types of avoidance that people might engage in instead of facing their situation or working to improve it. Some patients avoid talking about their feelings of self-hatred, but as Marsha Linehan states, "Avoidance of suffering leads to worse suffering." Many people with self-hatred are also convinced that their feelings won't change. This is untrue! There is significant research that shows that simply acknowledging and identifying negative emotions can reduce their impact and help you begin to change. Finally, comparisons get in the way of working on self-hatred because they enable people to justify their negative feelings about themselves. If comparisons feed your self-hatred, self-compassion can help you stop the cycle.

Praise doesn't help people overcome self-hatred, even when it comes from people they care about. Self-hatred makes it difficult for people to believe that others have positive thoughts about them, so accepting praise feels like accepting a lie. Compliments feel like they are given out of pity instead of sincerity. Praise feels undeserved. Positive affirmations may work somewhat, but their effects are short lived.

Key Definitions and Concepts

- **Avoidance:** Behaviors that show up when a person won't or refuses to enter into an experience of situation. It is a natural coping mechanism that often works in the short term by providing immediate relief, yet it has long-term consequences because the person never truly learns how to deal with the avoided situation. There are different types of avoidance:
  - **Situational avoidance:** Staying away from people, places, activities, and situations that cause a person distress. This is the most common type of avoidance.
  - **Somatic avoidance:** Staying away from physical sensations, including situations that cause physical distress like anxiety or stress.
  - **Cognitive avoidance:** Distracting oneself from thoughts or memories that are negative or hurtful.
  - **Protective avoidance:** Common in people with OCD, this includes engaging in behaviors that are seen as guarding against distress or perceived danger.
  - **Substitution avoidance:** Instead of facing a situation that causes suffering, a person engages in a different behavior to avoid negative feelings.
  - **Escape:** Leaving a situation when it becomes uncomfortable.
- **Cognitive dissonance:** The feeling that arises when a person holds two seemingly contradictory ideas or opinions. It can be very uncomfortable to acknowledge that both are correct.
- **Conditional worth:** Praise that focuses on innate qualities or inflated achievement, signaling that you are only valued because of those traits or accomplishments.
- **Evaluation anxiety:** Anxious feelings that arise when a person feels they are being evaluated, either positively or negatively.

Chapter 12 Warmup Activity: What Are Your Biggest Obstacles?

To begin to overcome your self-hatred, you need to face your obstacles. Consider the obstacles discussed in Chapter 12 of *I Hate Myself* and complete the following table.

Obstacle	Do You Experience This?	How and When Does It Emerge?
Avoidance		
Certainty that it can't change		
Comparisons		
Failure to accept praise		

Avoidance and Escape

In therapy, avoidance behaviors are the actions you take to prevent experiencing distressing thoughts, emotions, memories, or situations, usually by not entering, discussing, or confronting what feels upsetting. Escape behaviors are behaviors you take to leave or discontinue a situation after the distress has already begun, often seeking immediate relief from the discomfort or anxiety, and this is where dangerous and maladaptive behaviors like self-injury might show up because self-injury and other destructive behaviors can lead to rapid and temporary relief from emotional pain. Let's look at these behaviors more specifically.

- **Avoidance behaviors:** Avoidance means keeping away from discussing certain activities, people, places, or topics to reduce perceived danger or anxiety. For instance, you might say: "I don't go to therapy sessions where I might have to talk about abuse or my abuser." You might also say, "I don't want to talk about self-hatred because I have to think about the pain of my childhood." Common examples in therapy include not completing your therapist's assigned homework, such as not doing some of the worksheets in this book, or not sharing your emotions, or refusing to process some of the painful reminders and memories of your early childhood.
- **Escape behaviors:** Again, escape involves reacting by leaving or disengaging from distress once it has started, for instance, "I walk out of group or therapy if I feel overwhelmed." Other common examples in therapy include suddenly shutting down emotionally during a difficult topic or jumping to a completely other topic as soon as discomfort arises.

Activity 12.1 in this workbook chapter addresses avoidance and escape.

Comparison

One of the least helpful, and perhaps even aggravating, behaviors you can exhibit when you have self-hatred is to compare yourself to others. And yet the modern world, through social media and endless TV shows, tells you that you are not enough. Comparing yourself to others can worsen your self-hatred because it often highlights your perceived shortcomings, triggers feelings of inadequacy, and leads to destructive patterns of envy, shame, and negative self-talk. Frequent comparison fixates attention on where you fall short, magnifying your sense of not measuring up to others and eroding your self-worth and self-acceptance.

And yet there is a way that comparisons can help! For some with lived experience, the exercise of comparing themselves to historical figures who have done some truly terrible things can help put your experience and sense of self into a bigger perspective. Many people with core self-hatred can believe that they are the worst person ever and feel as if the world would be better off had they never been born. Because they are so consumed by their self-hatred, they cannot see their innate worth, and nor can they see that they are not even anywhere close to how awful other human beings have been in the past or even are, in the present.

Comparison fuels self-hatred in many ways. These are some of the most common:

- **Focus on flaws:** Constantly measuring your worth against others leads you to overlook your own strengths and achievements, and instead, obsess over what you lack. This selective attention reinforces beliefs of being "less than" and unworthy.
- **Negative self-talk:** Social comparison often causes an internal dialogue of self-criticism—"Why can't I be like them?"—which increases self-loathing, persistent dissatisfaction, and a cycle of shame.
- **Perfectionism pressure:** Seeing others' curated successes can push you to set unrealistic standards for yourself. This is what often happens when you watch the highly scripted and expertly produced social media videos, and then, when you can't meet unrealistic standards, self-blame and feelings of failure intensify.
- **Distorted reality:** Social media and public personas highlight only idealized moments. Comparing yourself to these highlight reels creates unfair standards, making everyday struggles seem unacceptable and deepening self-hatred when life doesn't measure up.

These mechanisms are summarized in Table 12.1.

Table 12.1 Common Comparison Mechanisms

Mechanism of Comparison	Effect on Self-Hatred
Focus on perceived deficits	Increased self-loathing and inadequacy
Negative internal commentary	Persistent self-criticism, shame
Unrealistic expectations	Perfectionism, belief of personal failure
Social media exposure	Amplified envy, distorted self-worth

Comparison can have serious psychological consequences. Increased anxiety, depression, and chronic self-doubt are common outcomes of toxic comparison with others. Self-hatred becomes your default mode as comparison activates persistent negative emotions such as jealousy, frustration, and hopelessness.

Praise

If you have experienced self-hatred, you will have people in your life who want to praise you as a way of challenging how you see yourself. What you might have felt and what they don't know is that praise can feel toxic or uncomfortable to people with self-hatred. Compliments and praise can clash with your internal beliefs, provoking anxiety, mistrust, and even increased self-loathing rather than reassurance. Why might praise feel toxic?

- **Cognitive dissonance:** When praise contradicts entrenched self-hatred, it may feel false, triggering discomfort or suspicion—"If they only knew who I really am, they wouldn't say that." This disconnect can magnify feelings of being misunderstood or unworthy.
- **Conditional worth:** Praise that focuses on innate qualities, for instance, a statement like "You're so smart!" or inflated achievement can reinforce fears of conditional acceptance—feeling that you're loved only when you're successful, worsening shame after perceived failures or setbacks.
- **Evaluation anxiety:** Receiving praise is also a form of interpersonal evaluation, which can heighten anxiety and self-consciousness if you already feel defective or "broken" inside.
- **Internal critic activation:** Compliments may activate your inner critic, with your mind quickly discounting or arguing against positive feedback. You might say things like: "They must be lying. I don't deserve this," reinforcing cycles of shame and distrust of kindness.

And there is research that supports this. One study shows that what the researchers call "person praise," or praised focused on traits rather than process or effort, can lower self-worth and future motivation, especially in those with low self-esteem. Another study shows that compliments may trigger more shame and avoidance in people with self-hatred, undermining rather than bolstering well-being. Activity 12.4 can help you tackle issues you might have with praise.

The Role of Core Beliefs

This section explores why self-hatred is so difficult to treat, the limitations of traditional therapies, and the importance of directly targeting core beliefs, avoidance, and comparison. It is designed to help you reflect on your experiences, identify barriers, and begin to challenge entrenched patterns of self-loathing.

To review, overcoming longstanding self-hatred is difficult because it is deeply rooted in early life experiences—reinforced by negative self-talk, societal pressures, and sometimes trauma—often becoming ingrained over years as part of core identity and beliefs. These beliefs are not simply fleeting thoughts but persistent, habitual patterns that fundamentally shape one's view of self and the world.

There are four key reasons for this difficulty:

1. **Early formation and reinforcement:** Self-hatred often starts with childhood experiences such as criticism, neglect, abuse, or invalidation. These messages become internalized as absolute truths and shape core self-beliefs, making reversal slow and challenging. Core self-hatred has the quality of feeling as if is a part of the self, like gender identity. Further, societal and cultural standards around worth, success, and beauty can reinforce feelings of inadequacy and perpetuate self-loathing.
2. **Habitual negative self-talk:** Persistent negative self-talk functions like a corrosive destructive psychological force—critical thoughts become automatic, habitual, and difficult to interrupt, forming a powerful internal narrative. Then, shame and self-hatred feed off each other, creating a cycle in which critical self-judgments continually reinforce emotional pain and vice versa. Throughout the book mindfulness is a key practice and in particular mindfulness of self-hatred thoughts. Habitual negative self-talk is the opposite of mindfulness, or mindlessness. Habits and mindlessness are closely connected because habits are behaviors that, through repetition, become automatic and are often carried out with little conscious awareness or intentional thought. When a behavior is performed frequently in stable contexts, it transitions from a mindful action, an action requiring attention, to a "mindless" one—executed on

autopilot. There are times when mindlessness is necessary. Having to deeply and mindfully ponder the nature of a red traffic light makes little sense, and automatically stopping makes more sense. On the other hand, there is a significant risk to mindlessness when it comes to habitual self-hatred. The first is stagnation and inflexibility in that mindless repetition can stifle personal growth, reduce responsiveness to change, and lock you into unhelpful and maladaptive self-perceptions. The second is that breaking mindless habits and developing healthier ones involves bringing mindful attention to automatic behaviors, noticing triggers, and intentionally choosing new actions, and mindlessness automaticity is inconsistent with mindful action.

3. **Emotional impact and vicious cycles:** Self-hatred is closely tied to mental health diagnoses, as reviewed in Chapter 7—especially borderline personality disorder, depression, and eating disorders—where it both results from and worsens symptoms, locking individuals into downward spirals of shame, isolation, and hopelessness. Self-hatred can even feel familiar or safe, paradoxically giving a sense of control amidst uncertainty, making it difficult to relinquish even when it is distressing.
4. **Resistance to compassion and change:** Chronic self-loathing erodes self-worth and can create strong resistance to self-compassion, making kind self-talk and positive interventions feel false or impossible at first. Emotional setbacks and triggers can quickly reactivate entrenched patterns, even after progress is made.

To start to address these barriers, the first step is to become aware of them. One way to start is to first identify your core beliefs. Core beliefs are deeply held, fundamental ideas about yourself, others, and the world that shape how you interpret experiences and respond to life's challenges. These beliefs develop early in life and act as mental filters, like looking at the world through dark or rose-colored glasses, lenses through which all situations are viewed, influencing emotions, behavior, and decision-making.

As stated, they relate to three domains: (a) the self—thoughts such as "I am unlovable" or "I am capable"; (b) to others—thoughts like "People are trustworthy" or "People will hurt me"; or (c) to the world—statements like "Life is unfair" or "The world is safe."

Core beliefs operate below conscious awareness, guiding automatic thoughts and shaping emotional and behavioral responses—even if not explicitly recognized. Because most of us are unaware of our core beliefs, this is where the practice of mindfulness is so key. Harmful core beliefs can create negative patterns of thinking, such as persistent self-doubt or cynicism, or as it pertains to this book, self-hatred. However, helpful core beliefs boost resilience and optimism.

Activity 12.1: Comparisons

Identify three of the most hated people in history. For each, identify three characteristics or actions that justify their poor reputation, then answer the questions that follow the table.

Historical Figure	Characteristics or Actions

1. Compare yourself to these people. In what ways are you similar?

2. What does this reflection do to your sense of how "bad" or "flawed" you are?

Activity 12.2: Avoidance and Escape

Identify ways you avoid or escape from thinking about self-hatred.

1. What situations, thoughts, or feelings do you avoid when experiencing self-hatred?

2. Have you avoided talking to your therapist about it?

3. When you do think or talk about it in therapy, do you use any escape behaviors such as changing topics or shutting down?

4. What about when you are not in therapy; do you use escape behaviors such as distraction, substance use, self-injury, or social withdrawal?

5. How does avoidance of addressing impact your progress in therapy or self-growth?

Activity 12.3: The Role of Comparison

In this next worksheet, you can explore how comparison to others (or to your past/future self) fuels self-hatred. This exercise is different from and yet builds on, the exercise in Activity 12.1 in that there are realistic comparisons in everyday life, but when you consider yourself the worst person ever, the activity of comparing yourself to the worst people ever puts your reflection into perspective.

1. Do you compare yourself to others?

2. Who are the people you compare yourself to? Are they people in your life? Social media influencers? Celebrities?

____

____

____

____

3. How do these comparisons make you feel?

____

____

____

____

4. Can you identify moments when comparison triggered self-loathing? Write them here.

____

____

____

____

Activity 12.4: The Problem with Praise

Reflect on your reactions to praise and positive feedback.

1. How do you feel when someone praises you?

____

____

____

____

2. Do you believe them or dismiss their words?

3. Do you feel that they "have to" say nice things, particularly if praise is coming from a friend or family member? Why or why not?

4. When you praise others, is your praise genuine? Why or why not?

5. What would it take for you to accept praise as genuine?

6. Finally, because you might find praise to be unhelpful, let the person who is praising you know that you are working on developing a healthier sense of self and that receiving praise is not helpful. Recognize the intent behind the praise.

Activity 12.5: Direct Communication

When the people around you use praise with the intention of reducing your self-hatred, you can let them know that being praised is not helpful. You might suggest what might be helpful instead; aim for honesty and specificity while respecting both your perspective and the other person's intentions. Use this activity to organize your thoughts so you can communicate clearly.

1. **Frame the conversation:** Recognize the intention behind the praise and that it is appreciated even if it is not helpful. Identify the people with whom you would want to have this conversation. (Example: "I really appreciate that you want to encourage me, but I actually find praise unhelpful.")

   ____

   ____

   ____

   ____

2. **Explain why praise isn't helpful:** You might want to share how praise affects you. Specificity helps:

- "When I hear things like 'good job' or general compliments, it sometimes feels like pressure, or it doesn't tell me much about what was actually useful or effective."
- "Sometimes praise makes me feel awkward, or as if my effort is being seen in a way that doesn't match how I experienced it."

   ____

   ____

   ____

   ____

3. **Suggest alternatives:** Offer suggestions for what kind of feedback, acknowledgment, or interaction would be more positive:

- "Instead of praise, it helps me more if you give me specific feedback about what worked or what could be adjusted next time."

- "I prefer neutral acknowledgments, like noting that something was completed, or specific suggestions for improvement."

4. Promote open dialogue: Welcome clarification and conversation: "Is that okay with you? I'd be happy to talk more about what kind of feedback helps me stay motivated and supported."

Being open and descriptive helps the other person adjust their support in a way that matches your needs, rather than relying on default expressions of praise.

Activity 12.6: Identifying My Core Beliefs

List your core beliefs—both general and personal. Reflect on how they were shaped by your experiences.

- What are some beliefs you hold about yourself, others, and the world?

- Which beliefs feel helpful, and which feel harmful?

- Can you trace any beliefs back to specific experiences or relationships?

Fill in the following table; use your own core beliefs unless the ones listed are consistent with yours.

Type of Belief	**Example and Your Belief**	**Helpful or Harmful?**	**Origin/Experience**
Universal norm	"Murder is wrong."	Helpful	Society
Social/ practical norm	"I should show up to work on time."	Helpful	Society
Personal core belief	"I am unlovable."	Harmful	Childhood criticism

Harmful core belief	"I'll never be good enough."	Harmful	School comparisons

Activity 12.7: Challenging the Certainty of Self-Hatred

This activity challenges the certainty of these beliefs to erode their hold on your mind. It is as if self-hatred were a sandcastle that you believed was solid. Let the practices in this workbook erode the sands of certainty. Reflect on the belief that your self-hatred is permanent or unchangeable.

- Do you believe that you were born self-hating?

____

____

____

____

- Do you believe your self-hatred is a fixed part of you?

____

____

____

____

- What evidence supports that self-hatred is a fixed part of you?

____

____

____

____

- What evidence contradicts this belief? Take your time to answer this question honestly.

____

____

____

____

- Imagine your future self, looking back at you today: Would you judge yourself as harshly as you do now, knowing all that you do now?

____

____

____

____

- Can you imagine a person going through everything you have gone through and being mean to your younger self?

____

____

____

____

Key Points

- Many therapists don't ask about self-hatred during intake, and patients often avoid discussing it due to shame, creating an invisible barrier to treatment.
- Avoidance behaviors (refusing to discuss feelings) and escape behaviors (leaving situations when uncomfortable) perpetuate suffering by preventing healing.
- Comparison to others amplifies self-hatred by highlighting perceived shortcomings, though comparing yourself to truly harmful people can provide perspective.
- Praise often feels toxic to people with self-hatred due to cognitive dissonance, triggering the inner critic rather than building self-worth.
- Self-hatred is difficult to overcome because it's formed early, reinforced by habitual negative self-talk, tied to identity, and resistant to compassion.

Chapter 13

Reflections of Therapists

Chapter Summary

Many therapists are trained in the types of approaches that can help people with self-hatred. In Chapter 13 of *I Hate Myself*, I include reflections from therapists working with clients in three different therapy contexts. These stories represent larger trends, including that many therapists recognize that their clients experience self-loathing and how it can affect daily life. Despite this, many therapists don't ask their clients about self-hatred and are uncertain about how to treat it. This can understandably seem discouraging, but many therapists also understand the types of therapies and approaches that can help people with self-loathing.

The first step should be to talk with your therapist so they understand the kind of care you need. Through that conversation, you'll also learn whether they seem to be a good fit.

Key Definitions and Concepts

- **Therapeutic relationship:** The way a therapist and client interact, including whether the client feels there is enough trust and rapport to discuss whatever they want. The type of therapy you need depends on the underlying issues that bring you to therapy, so it's essential to find a therapist who aligns with your specific needs.
- **Psychotherapy:** Mental health treatment that involves talking with a trained therapist to address emotional challenges, behavioral issues, or other mental health conditions.

This chapter will explore more about why therapists don't ask about self-hatred, and why therapy may not have worked up to now in reducing your feelings of self-loathing.

Chapter 13 Warmup Activity: When Therapy and Self-Compassion Haven't Worked

Think about your current or previous therapy experiences or self-help strategies that didn't help your self-hatred. Review your answers with your therapist to ensure you share an understanding of your experience so far.

1. Why types of therapies have you tried?

 ____

 ____

 ____

 ____

2. What kind of therapy are you currently in?

 ____

 ____

 ____

 ____

3. What other approaches have you tried (e.g., self-affirmations, self-compassion exercises)?

 ____

 ____

 ____

 ____

4. Why do you think these didn't work for you?

____

____

____

____

5. Did any of these attempts make your self-hatred worse? How?

____

____

____

____

6. Where there any interventions that did help, even if just a little? Which ones?

____

____

____

____

The activities at the end of this chapter dig deeper into your current therapy.

Why Therapists Don't Ask About Self-Hatred

This workbook chapter highlights the surprising reality that many therapists are not trained to ask about or directly address self-hatred, despite its prevalence and profound impact. The following worksheets are designed to help you and your therapist open up the conversation, recognize barriers, and begin to collaboratively address self-hatred in your therapy. Generally speaking, therapists don't bring up the topic of self-hatred for two reasons: The first is that clients don't bring it up as an issue to address in therapy, and the second is that therapists aren't trained to ask about it. There are some other reasons why self-hatred is not brought up.

Activity 13.1, at the end of this chapter, may be a fun one for you as a client, because it asks the therapist to reflect on why they have not addressed your self-hatred!

Why Therapy Might Not Have Worked So Far

Next, let's review reasons why your therapy may not have worked for self-hatred. The most common reason has to do with it not being a topic of therapy, and this can be because you never brought it up, or because your therapist never brought it up, as discussed. However there are other reasons: There might not be a good fit with your therapist, you and your therapist may not have set up clear goals, there might be a mismatch between the treatment type and your needs, there may be therapist-related problems, you may have severe or acute symptoms needing more intensive care, and there may be other external barriers to progress, for instance demanding work, family or school pressures.

Let's look deeper into the circumstances where psychotherapy is less effective. If you are struggling in therapy, consider the following factors:

- **Poor therapeutic relationship:** When you think about your relationships with your therapist, do you have trust, have rapport, and feel safe to discuss whatever you want? Or is there a mismatch in therapeutic style?
- **Unclear or unrealistic goals:** Therapy may stagnate if you and your therapist did not set clear goals, do not agree on the goals for your therapy, or have unrealistic expectations about your progress. Have you and your therapist set clear goals?
- **Therapist factors:** Perhaps your therapist did not do a proper assessment of your needs when they completed the initial intake or is very inflexible in their approach. Perhaps they lack empathy, or have inadequate skills to help you, or avoid addressing important problems. Are there any therapist factors that might be interfering?
- **Severity of symptoms:** You may have symptoms so severe (e.g., psychosis, suicidality, intense trauma) that weekly therapy is insufficient, and you may require a higher level of care, medication, or a more specialized approach. Is addressing self-hatred once a week a viable approach, or do you need more intensive treatment to address other severe symptoms?
- **Inappropriate treatment type:** Success depends on the right match between the therapy approach and your problems; some treatment

Table 13.1 Factors Associated with Psychotherapy Failure

Factor	Example Impact
Poor therapeutic relationship	Lack of trust, feeling judged, withdrawal
Unclear or unrealistic goals	Disappointment, lack of direction
Therapist problems (skills, empathy, ethics)	Lack of empathy, early termination of therapy
Severity of symptoms	Requires medication or intensive care
Being disengaged	Missed sessions, no progress
Wrong treatment approach/type	Symptoms persist, frustration
External/life barriers	Stress, lack of time, physical illness

modalities may fit certain issues poorly, for instance exposure and response prevention (ERP) is not the approach for borderline personality disorder, and group therapy may be harmful for very vulnerable or mismatched individuals. Does the treatment type and approach identify the ways in which it will help with your struggles?

- **External factors:** Life circumstances—such as family crises or physical illness—may make it difficult to address self-hatred. Is anything outside of your own mental state interfering with or aggravating your ability to do the work?

Table 13.1 summarizes these factors and the type of impact they can have. Thinking about all these factors, complete Activity 13.1.

Barriers to Addressing Self-Hatred in Therapy

As mentioned repeatedly throughout this workbook, one barrier to tackling self-hatred is if your therapist does not bring it up, but another barrier is if you yourself don't bring it up. Barriers to bringing up self-hatred in therapy include your feeling intense shame, fear of judgment, internalized stigma, emotional vulnerability, distrust, and the tendency to feel unworthy or undeserving of support. These obstacles may prevent you from honestly disclosing self-hatred, despite it being a major driver of emotional distress.

Here are some key barriers, which are also summarized in Table 13.2:

- **Shame and stigma:** Deep feelings of shame, embarrassment, or perceived failure can make self-hatred too painful or humiliating to discuss. You may worry that your therapist will judge you or think less of you.
- **Feeling undeserving:** Many struggling with self-hatred believe they don't deserve help or treatment, leading them to minimize or hide their inner experience.
- **Vulnerability and trust issues:** Fear of being vulnerable, rejected, or misunderstood may stop you from opening up about self-loathing, especially if your history includes emotional neglect or relational trauma.
- **Defensive coping:** Self-hatred can function as a protective defense—you may use self-hatred to avoid talking about it to escape deeper feelings of pain, risk of shame, or further emotional harm.
- **Mental health system challenges:** Because at the time of this writing, there are not many therapists who actively tackle self-hatred, structural issues, such as untrained therapists, negative professional attitudes, and long waiting lists for specialists like DBT therapists, make it harder to access support for self-hatred and related struggles.

Which of these resonate with you, and how do these barriers manifest in your therapy?

Table 13.2 Summary of Barriers

Barrier	How It Impedes Discussing Self-Hatred
Shame and stigma	Fear of judgment, humiliation, or exposure
Feeling undeserving	Belief that you are not worthy of care or help
Vulnerability	Fear of rejection/relational wounds
Defensive coping	Avoidance of pain and risk
Systemic/access issues	Hard to reach qualified, supportive providers

Activity 13.1: Interview Your Therapist

Ask your therapist if the following list items are pertinent to their therapeutic relationship with you. Take time to discuss and write down notes based on their answers.

1. **Your therapist fears overwhelming you:** This is also the concept of treating you as fragile, as if you can't deal with the topic. Self-hatred is frequently tied to deeply rooted shame, trauma, and vulnerability. Therapists may avoid direct confrontation with these feelings until the you have developed enough coping resources and trust, because they worry that they might retraumatize or destabilize you.

Ask your therapist: "Are you afraid of emotionally overwhelming me?"
Answer:

____

____

____

____

2. **Your therapist worries that you will become defensive or that you are not ready:** You might use self-hatred as a defense strategy to control rejection or avoid further emotional risk. It is possible that you might shut down if your therapist challenges your defenses, which can lead you to not being as engaged in therapy as you could be.

Ask your therapist: "Are you afraid that I will become defensive or that I am not ready to do this work?"
Answer:

____

____

____

____

3. **Your therapist feels discomfort:** If you have strong emotions and experiences such as self-hatred, this can be unsettling for your therapist, resulting in their avoidance, their rapid topic-changing, or a tendency for them to redirect the conversation toward less distressing material.

Ask your therapist: "Are you uncomfortable bringing up the topic?"
Answer:

____

____

____

____

4. **Your therapist considers pacing and process:** Because self-hatred is not a standard target for therapy, your therapist might prioritize skill building, understanding, and your building self-acceptance. To do this, they might insist on working at a slower pace, choosing not to name or focus directly on "self-hatred" until you feel safer, more stable, and able to tolerate painful self-awareness and emotions.

Ask your therapist: "Are you spending too much time on other aspects of therapy and not focusing at all on my self-hatred?"
Answer:

____

____

____

____

5. **Your therapist respects your defenses:** Sometimes, your defenses—for instance, self-hatred—can help you survive emotionally, because you set very low expectations for yourself—so low that you can't be disappointed. Your therapist might honor this defense until you develop healthier self-protective mechanisms, which can be cultivated to allow defenses to dissolve with time rather than being forcefully dismantled. Healthier defense mechanisms, such as humor and altruism, allow you to manage emotions productively and foster growth or connection, rather than causing you to be avoidant, to use distortion, or to cause you harm.

Ask your therapist: "Are you overly validating my self-hatred?"

Answer:

Activity 13.2: Acceptance Versus Change: My Experience in Therapy

Reflect on your experiences with acceptance-focused and change-focused therapies.

1. Is your therapy a change-focused therapy such as CBT. If you don't know, you can ask your therapist.

2. Is your therapy an acceptance-focused therapy, such as psychoanalysis or talk therapy? Write the approach here.

3. Have you felt validated and understood in therapy? Why or why not?

4. Did it help to address your self-hatred? Why do you think that is?

5. Have you been encouraged to "change your thinking" or "practice self-love"? If so, how?

6. How did that feel?

7. Have any approaches felt supportive? If so, which ones, and how did they feel supportive?

8. Have any approaches or situations felt invalidating? If so, which ones and how?

9. Can you let your therapist know directly that their approach feels invalidating? Why or why not?

Activity 13.3: Therapist Assessment: Self-Hatred Inquiry

This activity is for your therapist to complete. *Reflect on your clinical practice using these questions* (adapted from Chapter 13 in *I Hate Myself*).

1. *Do you see patients who have disclosed self-hatred? What percentage of your caseload is affected?*

2. *Do you routinely ask about self-hatred during initial assessments?*

3. *How does self-hatred manifest in your patients (e.g., hopelessness, avoidance, anger, perfectionism)?*

4. *How has self-hatred impacted your patients' lives and treatment progress?*

____

____

____

____

5. *How does patient disclosure of self-hatred impact you?*

____

____

____

____

6. *Is your tendency to try to convince your patient that they shouldn't hate themselves, or to point out all the things that they have in their lives as reasons why they shouldn't hate themselves?*

____

____

____

____

7. *Have you directly addressed self-hatred in therapy? What were the challenges or successes?*

____

____

____

____

Activity 13.4: Identifying Barriers to Discussing Self-Hatred

Explore what makes it hard to talk about self-hatred in therapy.

1. Do you feel that you deserve therapy or deserve to be helped with self-hatred? Why or why not?

____

____

____

____

2. Have you found it difficult to find someone who knows anything about self-hatred and how to treat it? Who? What have you learned?

____

____

____

____

3. Are you worried your therapist will judge you or think less of you? Why?

____

____

____

____

4. Are you worried that they will not know how to help? Why?

____

____

____

____

5. Have you ever avoided bringing up self-hatred because it felt destabilizing or overwhelming? Why?

____

____

____

____

6. Would it make you feel vulnerable if you talked about it, as if you are exposing a very dark side of yourself? Or you believe that your therapist will "realize" that you truly are an awful person?

____

____

____

____

7. What would make it safer or easier to bring up these feelings in therapy?

____

____

____

____

If you have overcome the barriers to your not talking about it and your therapist not bringing it up, what next? This next worksheet includes ideas for creating a treatment plan.

Activity 13.5: Therapist–Client Collaboration Plan

Use this worksheet together with your therapist to set goals for addressing self-hatred.

- How will self-hatred be assessed?

____

____

____

____

- Are you both committed to working on self-hatred?

- What specific aspects of self-hatred do you want to work on?

- What skills or strategies (e.g., exposure tasks, mindfulness, self-compassion) might help?

- Will your therapist assign regular homework? And are you committed to doing it?

- How will you and your therapist check in on progress and adjust the plan as needed?

Not all your work will be addressed in a therapy session, and there are many things that you can do at home or in non-therapy time to continue the work of building yourself up and eroding your self-hatred. Further, you must continue to tackle the things that make self-hatred hard to discuss.

Key Points

- Many therapists recognize self-hatred but don't ask about it directly, often due to lack of training, fear of overwhelming clients, or discomfort with the topic.
- Therapy may fail when there's a poor therapeutic relationship, unclear goals, inappropriate treatment type, therapist skill gaps, or severe symptoms needing intensive care.
- Barriers to discussing self-hatred include shame, feeling undeserving of help, fear of vulnerability, and defensive coping mechanisms.
- Balance between acceptance-focused (validation) and change-focused (skills) approaches is crucial—too much of either can feel invalidating or overwhelming.
- Direct therapist–client collaboration on self-hatred treatment plans, including specific goals, skills, and homework, is essential for progress.

Chapter 14

Advice from Those with Lived Experience

Chapter Summary

Many people with self-hatred don't even realize that it's something that needs to be addressed in therapy. It just feels like a part of them. Many of the patients I've talked to were surprised when I asked about self-hatred because most therapists don't bring it up. Once they ask about self-hatred in therapy, they are able to work to reduce its power.

The concept of a future you can help you address self-loathing because it puts you in the mindset to visualize your success, which allows you to reconsider what your future looks like. Your future needs you! If you are able to imagine a future version of yourself that has more self-compassion, you can find motivation in the present that will help you become that future person. Even if you don't feel like that person today, the small steps you take today, tomorrow, and the next day will help you become your imagined future self.

Another thing that can help you with self-loathing is to practice self-acceptance. This is when you practice self-compassion and learn to accept your suffering. In doing so, you can recognize that your suffering has caused your self-hatred, but that you can still appreciate the positive parts of life. It is possible for the good and bad to come together.

There are many other techniques and strategies that people with lived experience of self-hatred find helpful:

- Do something you love doing every day, even if just for a few minutes.
- Notice the moments when the feeling of self-hatred changes.
- Compare yourself to historically loathed people.
- Identify with the qualities you admire in people you admire.

- Dismiss the bullies and tormentors of your past.
- Realize that self-hatred was learned.
- Strive for independence.
- Complete a list of pros and cons.
- Focus on the right side of storytelling versus the wrong side of storytelling.
- Accept the current moment.
- Practice core self-compassion.
- Be honest with yourself about the value of the work you do.
- Talk about self-hatred in therapy.
- Check the "facts" that support your conclusion of self-hatred.
- Tackle the fear of getting better.

Many of these are tied to concepts that can support a powerful shift in your perspective. For more information on these, refer to *I Hate Myself.*

Key Definitions and Concepts

- **Future you:** An imagined future self who has accomplished at least one of your goals.
- **Possible selves:** The concept that we all have many possible futures that are influenced by the choices we make each day.
- **Exposure:** The concept of exposure in therapy is where a person is gradually and safely confronted with a feared object, situation, or memory in a controlled environment to reduce fear and avoidance. It is a component of CBT and works by helping you learn that your fear responses are not harmful, and so retraining your brain to see any trigger as less threatening.

Chapter 14 Warmup Activity: Connecting With Your Future Self

Close your eyes and picture your future self, who, ideally, has learned to be more accepting of and kinder to themselves. If that feels too difficult or unimaginable, then picture a self who does at least one self-caring action for themselves every day.

1. What would they want you to know or do today?

___

___

___

___

2. Imagine yourself one year from now, having made progress in self-compassion. Write a letter from your future self, offering advice or encouragement for moments of self-doubt.

___

___

___

___

When struggling, revisit this letter or visualization to remind yourself that acceptance is a process, and your future self is cheering you on.

Find What Works for You

An exercise that has worked for those with lived experience is that of connecting with their future self. Meeting your future self can guide you toward acceptance in the present by offering perspective, hope, and actionable wisdom, a wisdom that reframes how you relate to yourself now. Here's how this process works:

1. **Inspiration and encouragement:** Your future self, the person that you want to be a week, a month, or a year from now, does not want to be hating themselves. Visualizing and even talking to your future self, one that no longer hates themselves and instead has compassion for you today, helps you receive inspiration and encouragement for the challenges you face today. By imagining a wiser, more compassionate version of yourself, you can access guidance and reassurance that self-acceptance is possible—even if it feels distant right now.
2. **Clarity on what truly matters:** Connecting with your future self allows you to clarify your core values and long-term goals. This perspective helps

you see beyond your current struggles or self-judgments, focusing instead on the bigger picture of who you want to become. When you know what your future self values, it becomes easier to accept your present self as a work in progress, rather than a finished product. Your future self does not value self-hatred. Be honest with yourself, is self-hatred truly a value of yours today?

3. **Positive impact on present choices:** Imagine your future self writing you a letter. Can you write that letter? Research shows that building a relationship with your future self can positively influence your current decisions, making it easier to choose self-kindness and acceptance over self-criticism. When you see yourself as someone who is growing and evolving toward that person in the future, you're more likely to treat yourself with patience and compassion in the present.
4. **Encouragement to take small, accepting steps:** Imagining your future self doesn't require envisioning a perfect, completely self-loving distant version of you. Even picturing yourself being a little bit kinder, a little less harsh on yourself a few months from now can help you identify small, manageable steps you can take now to move toward acceptance. This approach emphasizes progress over perfection and helps you accept where you are today as a valid part of your journey.
5. **Embodying self-acceptance:** Imagine that you could be in the mind of your future self and that you could know how they think, feel, and act. Imagine that person being kinder to you the way that you would be kinder to the child that was hurt. You can practice embodying qualities like self-acceptance and self-compassion right now. This experiential exercise helps you feel what it's like to accept yourself, making it easier to bring up those feelings more regularly into your daily life and particularly when self-hatred is strong.

Mindfulness Practice

Earlier, you practiced mindfulness of past invalidation. Let's review the "describe" skill or practice of DBT mindfulness. The skill involves putting words to your observations and doing so without judgment or interpretations, focusing only on the facts of the situation, thoughts, or emotions. It means verbally labeling what you're experiencing, such as sensations or feelings, as simply sensations of feeling, to create a clear, factual record and gain distance from thoughts and emotions, preventing them from being mistaken for facts. For example, instead of believing the thought "I'm a worthless person," you might describe how the thought arose, for instance, "I made a mistake on a report at work and my boss looked disappointed, and I had the thought 'I am a worthless person'." Doing this separates the observation from interpretation and emotional distress.

Another mindfulness practice is the 5-4-3-2-1 grounding technique, a practice that uses your five senses to help you manage anxiety and stress by focusing on connecting you to the present moment. Here is the practice:

- **5: See.** Look around and identify five things you can see in your immediate environment. Notice small details like colors, shapes, and textures.
- **4: Touch.** Find four things you can feel or touch. This might be the fabric of your clothes, the texture of your chair, or the solidity of the floor under your feet.
- **3: Hear.** Listen for and name three distinct sounds. You can focus on things you might typically tune out, like the hum of an appliance, the ticking of a clock, or distant traffic.
- **2: Smell.** Identify two different things you can smell. If you can't smell anything immediately, you can sniff your shirt, lotion, or a food item if there is one.
- **1: Taste.** Focus on one thing you can taste. This could be the lingering flavor of coffee, the inside of your mouth, or a sip of water.

Activity 14.1: Mindful Awareness of the Present (DBT/ACT)

Try grounding yourself with the 5-4-3-2-1 mindfulness practice. Write down your answers here.

5: See. Identify five things you can see in your immediate environment. Notice small details like colors, shapes, and textures.

____

____

____

____

4: Touch. Find four things you can feel or touch.

3: Hear. Listen for and name three distinct sounds. You can focus on things you might typically tune out, like the hum of an appliance, the ticking of a clock, or distant traffic.

2: Smell. Identify two different things you can smell. If you can't smell anything immediately, you can sniff your shirt, lotion, or a food item if there is one.

1: Taste. Focus on one thing you can taste. This could be the lingering flavor of coffee, the inside of your mouth, or a sip of water.

You can do this activity anytime you need to focus or calm yourself, or if your emotions become overwhelming. Your answers will be different each time because they connect you to your immediate environment.

Noticing Shifts in Self-Hatred

Nothing in the universe remains fixed. In dialectical behavior therapy (DBT), the concept of impermanence refers to the understanding that all emotions, thoughts, and experiences are temporary—sometimes they intensify and at other times they fade, but they always end. This is no different from the concept of constant change in the field of physics, which refers to the idea that the universe and all its physical phenomena are continuously evolving. Within every experience there are changes and fluctuations. If you think of a body of water, the surface is never completely flat; sometimes there are tiny ripples and at other times huge waves, but the water is never static. Similarly, it can feel as if self-hatred is constant, but it isn't. There will be times when you feel it more intensely and other times when it is less obvious even if it is there all the time. For some people with lieved experience, noticing these shifts can help. Try this next exercise.

A note for therapists: *Use these activities to open up direct conversations about self-hatred, assess its impact, and collaboratively develop treatment plans. Normalize the difficulty of discussing self-hatred and validate the client's experience. Integrate DBT, ACT, CBT, and mindfulness skills as appropriate, focusing on both acceptance and change.*

Activity 14.2: Noticing Shifts in Self-Hatred

Noticing shifts in self-hatred can remind you that it is a transient experience, not a permanent state. Answer the following questions to help yourself notice patterns in your feelings.

1. List situations when your self-hatred is strongest (e.g., after criticism, when you are alone, when you are comparing yourself to others).

 ____

 ____

 ____

 ____

2. List times when self-hatred is less intense (e.g., doing something you enjoy, helping others, being creative).

____

____

____

____

3. Now, list the people in your life or in your memory who intensify the feeling of self-hatred.

____

____

____

____

4. List the ones who lift you up and make you feel better about yourself.

____

____

____

____

5. Are there activities or situations that help reduce your self-hatred, even if briefly?

____

____

____

____

6. Do you have any choice in how you spend your time and or the people you choose to be with? Why or why not do you feel that way?

____

____

____

____

7. Do you choose situations that are more likely to lead to self-hatred because you do not believe that you deserve any better? Explain your answer.

____

____

____

____

8. Can you commit to spending a little more time with people who care about you and doing the things that make you feel better about yourself, and less time with the people who hurt you and doing the things that make you feel worse about yourself? What changes will you make?

____

____

____

____

Checking the Facts

Next is the DBT skill of Check the Facts. It is a useful skill that can help when emotions are running high and involves objectively examining the facts of a situation to determine if your emotional response is justified. It helps differentiate facts from interpretations and assumptions, which are often distorted by emotions, and aims to ensure emotions align with the reality of a situation rather than only your thoughts about it. Here's how it works:

1. **Identify the emotion and the event.** First, identify the emotion you want to examine and the specific event that triggered it.
2. **Describe the facts.** Describe the event using only your senses and objective observations, avoiding any judgments, assumptions, or emotional language. In other words, only describe what was actually said in a situation, and what was actually seen, and do so without judgment.
3. **Examine interpretations.** Look at your thoughts, interpretations, and assumptions about the event and identify any cognitive distortions such as

black-and-white thinking. Label each thought as a thought, each interpretation as an interpretation, and each assumption as an assumption.

4. **Consider other perspectives.** If you are making negative interpretations, think of other possible interpretations of the event to get a more balanced view. However, recognize that positive interpretations are also simply interpretations. The goal here is to aim for balance.
5. **Assess the threat.** For many people with self-hatred, paranoia and feeling threatened sets in very quickly when there is conflict. Determine if you are assuming a threat is present and assess its likelihood.
6. **Determine if the emotion fits.** Finally, using steps 1–5, evaluate whether the intensity of your emotion fits the actual facts.

Activity 14.3: Checking the Facts

Check the facts to help you ease strong negative emotions and ground your thoughts in a more objective experience.

1. Describe a recent spike in self-hatred.

____

____

____

____

2. What are the objective facts of the situation?

____

____

____

____

3. What are your interpretations, assumptions, or judgments?

____

____

____

____

4. Do your conclusions fit the facts, or are they driven by emotion?

____

____

____

____

Exposure (CBT and DBT)

Exposure-based tasks can play a transformative role in addressing self-hatred, particularly when that self-hatred is driven by internalized shame or fear of self-acceptance. In a way, self-hatred is almost like a fear of yourself, and for many people with fears, avoidance of the fear is common. When it comes to self-hatred, this might include avoiding things that expose you to yourself, such as avoiding mirrors, intimacy, receiving compliments, or being emotionally seen. Exposure tasks aim to desensitize you to these "triggers of self-disgust" and replace automatic self-attack with self-compassion.

Through gradual emotional exposure, you learn that confronting painful self-beliefs (e.g., "I'm worthless") does not lead to collapse or rejection but to insight and resilience. This builds new neural associations of safety and worthiness.

Activity 14.4: Exposure Tasks for Building Self-Efficacy

List small, achievable tasks that challenge your avoidance and build confidence.

1. What is one thing you could do this week that feels slightly uncomfortable but possible (e.g., expressing a preference, raising your hand in class, wearing clothes that fit)?

____

____

____

____

2. After completing the task, reflect:

   a. How did you feel before, during, and after?

   ____

   ____

   ____

   ____

   b. How did it challenge your beliefs about yourself?

   ____

   ____

   ____

   ____

   c. Can you acknowledge your own effort or pride in this accomplishment?

   ____

   ____

   ____

   ____

3. In therapy this week, did you notice any urge to avoid talking about self-hatred?

   ____

   ____

   ____

   ____

4. How did you address this?

   ____

   ____

   ____

   ____

5. Did you notice your therapist not bringing it up?

____

____

____

____

6. Did you address this directly with them?

____

____

____

____

Key Points

- Visualizing a compassionate future self who has overcome self-hatred provides inspiration, clarity on values, and motivation for present-day changes.
- Noticing when self-hatred shifts in intensity (stronger alone, weaker when engaged in meaningful activities) reveals it's transient, not permanent.
- Mindfulness practices can help manage overwhelming emotions and create present-moment awareness.
- Exposure tasks that gradually challenge avoidance (like receiving compliments or expressing preferences) build self-efficacy and resilience.

Chapter 15

Alternative Treatment Ideas

Chapter Summary

Because self-hatred hasn't been as researched as much as other mental health experiences, there is little evidence to date that it responds to any established treatments and approaches. Thinking out of the box, there are also some individual reports of recovery using alternative treatments, which I believe deserve additional study in recovery from self-loathing. These include disparate ideas like the use of psychedelics, focusing on the vagus nerve and heart rate variability (HRV), and eye movement desensitization and reprocessing (EMDR), as well as some concepts from acceptance and commitment therapy (ACT). This chapter contains fewer exercises than other chapters; however I include some research not included in the original book that continues to support the aforementioned approaches.

Key Definitions and Concepts

- **Psychedelic therapy:** Approaches that use substances that alter perception, mood, or cognitive processes for the treatment of mental health conditions like depression, PTSD, and anxiety. When used in a controlled clinical setting, these substances can create altered states of awareness that can help patients process past experiences.
- **Micro dosing:** Taking very low doses of psychedelic substances on a regular schedule. The goal is to enhance focus and well-being without the more extreme, hallucinogenic effects.
- **The vagus nerve:** The longest nerve in the body, acting as a "superhighway" that connects the brain to major organs like the heart, lungs, and digestive tract. It's a key part of the "rest and digest" system, controlling

involuntary functions like breathing, heart rate, and digestion, and it relays sensory information between the brain and the body.

- **Heart rate variability (HRV):** The slight variation in the time between each of your heartbeats. A higher HRV generally suggests that your body is well-rested and can effectively balance stress, while a lower HRV can indicate that you are stressed or tired.
- **Eye movement desensitization and reprocessing (EMDR):** A type of psychotherapy in which people recall a stressful event and use rapid eye movements and other techniques to reprogram the event in a way that makes it less traumatic.
- **Acceptance and commitment therapy (ACT):** A type of therapy that helps people accept difficult thoughts and feelings instead of fighting them, so they can take meaningful action toward what's important to them. Instead of trying to eliminate unwanted emotions, it teaches you to make room for them and commit to actions aligned with your personal values, fostering psychological flexibility to live a more meaningful life.

This chapter doesn't have a warm-up activity because the ideas and techniques require a degree of expert oversight. When you've completed reading Chapter 15 of *I Hate Myself* and this workbook material, you will be ready for the activities at the end of this chapter. There, you will also find complete references so you can see the research I've used to support the statements here.

Psychedelics

I included psychedelics in *I Hate Myself* because there is evidence that could support their therapeutic use. I do not endorse or reject their use. I simply believe more research is needed because people suffering from unrelenting self-loathing should have access to any effective treatments, so all avenues should be seriously explored. Before continuing, there are a few key points of caution:

- If you have bipolar disorder, psychedelics pose an additional risk because they are activating and can trigger a manic episode.

- Psychedelics come with risk, and there is no established level or dose recommended for self-hatred. If you are curious about psychedelics, consult a therapist who is trained in psychedelic-assisted psychotherapy.

In Chapter 1, we reviewed concepts related to, but different from, self-hatred. There are other forms of negative self-evaluation, such as self-criticism and self-blame. Another concept is *negative self-belief confidence*, a state of low self-esteem characterized by a lack of confidence due to negative thoughts and a poor self-image. This often leads to self-doubt, sensitivity to criticism, and difficulty accepting accomplishments. A recent study[1] found strong evidence for a relationship between decreases in negative self-belief confidence and increases in well-being in participants who were given psilocybin, which is a psychedelic derived from mushrooms.

This builds on previous research showing similar results on the beneficial effects of psilocybin on reducing negative self-concept. These results are promising; however, the studies are small, and more research is needed, but if you have self-hatred, it is certainly worth discussing with your therapist.

The Vagus Nerve and Heart Rate Variability (HRV)

HRV is the measure of the natural variation in time between each heartbeat. It's not about your average heart rate, but the slight fluctuations in the interval between beats, which is a healthy and normal phenomenon. Higher HRV indicates a flexible nervous system, one that can adapt to stress, while lower HRV can signal the body is under more stress.

The vagus nerve is the longest nerve in the body and acts like a "mind-body highway," connecting the brain to organs like the heart, lungs, and digestive system. It controls many involuntary functions, such as heart rate, breathing, and digestion, and helps regulate the body's rest state. By relaying information in both directions, it plays a critical role in maintaining physical and mental well-being. It

---

[1] Zeifman, R.J., Spriggs, M.J., Kettner, H. et al. From relaxed beliefs under psychedelics (REBUS) to revised beliefs after psychedelics (REBAS). *Sci Rep* 15, 3651 (2025). https://doi.org/10.1038/s41598-023-28111-3.

is the primary regulator of HRV, with a stronger vagal tone indicating a healthy vagus nerve, which directly correlates to higher HRV.

People with healthy minds and bodies typically have higher HRV, and those with certain mental health conditions, such as borderline personality disorder (BPD) and post-traumatic stress disorder (PTSD), have a lower HRV, meaning that they have a poorer response to stress.

Negative self-evaluation is significantly correlated with poor HRV; for instance, one study[2] found that high levels of self-critical rumination are linked to lower resting HRV, which predicts increased somatic symptom distress and poorer subjective well-being. Those with low HRV are more vulnerable to the negative psychological impacts of self-criticism, while higher HRV appears protective against distress related to ruminative self-criticism.

In another study,[3] those with poor self-esteem had lower HRV and greater difficulties in regulating emotions, impulsive behavior, and maintaining emotional clarity. Low HRV was associated with higher anxiety and difficulty inhibiting impulsive responses to negative feelings.

Then, researchers[4] found that poor acceptance of negative emotions—a hallmark of self-hatred—shows the strongest negative association with HRV. People who struggle to accept negative emotional states exhibit the lowest levels of HRV, reflecting diminished mental flexibility and increased vulnerability to mental illness.

---

[2] Kocsel, N., Köteles, F., Galambos, A., and Kökönyei, G. The interplay of self-critical rumination and resting heart rate variability on subjective well-being and somatic symptom distress: A prospective study. *J Psychosom Res* 152, 110676 (2022). https://doi.org/10.1016/j.jpsychores.2021.110676.

[3] Williams, D.P., Cash, C., Rankin, C. et al. Resting heart rate variability predicts self-reported difficulties in emotion regulation: A focus on different facets of emotion regulation. *Front Psychol* 6, 261 (2015). https://doi.org/10.3389/fpsyg.2015.00261.

[4] Visted, E., Sørensen, L., Osnes, B. et al. The association between self-reported difficulties in emotion regulation and heart rate variability: The salient role of not accepting negative emotions. *Front Psychol* 9; 8, 328 (2017). https://doi.org/10.3389/fpsyg.2017.00328.

By contrast, another study[5] shows that self-compassion is associated with higher HRV, suggesting greater adaptive capacity to manage negative mood states and stress. People high in self-compassion show the ability to flexibly regulate emotional responses.

Given that higher HRV is associated with better self-evaluation and lower HRV is associated with negative self-evaluation, here are some ways to improve your HRV.

- Routine physical activity—such as yoga, brisk walking, cycling, or swimming—can increase HRV. Exercise lowers stress hormones, enhances cardiovascular health, and improves mood, all of which help regulate HRV for mental resilience.
- Slow, deep breathing techniques, for instance breathing at six breaths per minute, as well as mindfulness practices and meditation, directly impact the vagus nerve and increases HRV and helping manage anxiety and negative self-focus.
- Getting seven to nine hours of regular, high-quality sleep per night is one of the most reliable ways to improve HRV. Consistent sleep supports autonomic nervous system balance, boosts emotional regulation, and reduces stress reactivity.

Can you commit to doing all of these on a regular basis as a way to improve HRV?

Eye Movement Desensitization Reprocessing (EMDR)

EMDR is a type of therapy that helps the brain process traumatic memories, so they are no longer as disturbing. It works by having you focus on a distressing memory while a therapist guides you through repetitive side-to-side eye movements, hand taps, or sounds to help the brain re-process the experience and "file"

[5] Luo, X., Qiao, L., and Che, X. Self-compassion modulates heart rate variability and negative affect to experimentally induced stress. *Mindfulness* 9, 1522–1528 (2018). https://doi.org/10.1007/s12671-018-0900-9.

it away properly. This helps to reduce the emotional power of the memory, so you no longer feel stuck in the past, and with this comes the reprocessing of the negative core self-beliefs that are associated with painful traumatic memories. EMDR is not a technique that you can do alone and you will need an EMDR certified therapist to guide you through it.

Acceptance and Commitment Therapy (ACT)

ACT is a type of psychotherapy that helps people deal with negative and unhelpful thoughts and feelings including self-hatred, low self-esteem, and self-criticism. It does so by teaching acceptance of yourself and encouraging actions that align with personal values. It focuses on living a meaningful life by increasing psychological flexibility, which is the ability to be present, accept difficult thoughts and feelings, and commit to actions that align with your personal values. Unlike some therapies that aim to eliminate negative thoughts, ACT encourages acceptance of these thoughts and focuses on taking committed action toward what is important to you, even when doing so is difficult.

These alternative ideas show significant promise as ways to tackle self-hatred. If the other ideas in the book are only partially helpful, add these activities, but make sure that you are working with someone experienced in the techniques.

Activity 15.1: Defusion Exercise

Defusion is the practice of not fusing with your thoughts. At times, it can feel as if you and your thoughts are fused together. In this practice, watch your thoughts drift. Take these steps to practice defusion:

1. Imagine your negative self-judgments (like "I'm not good enough") as words floating by on clouds.
2. Visualize each thought, place it on a cloud, and watch it drift away.

While you can do this anywhere, if the weather is nice, and you are able to, go outside. (This works best if there are clouds in the sky.) Rather than visualizing clouds, you can pick an actual cloud, attach the negative thought to it, and watch the cloud change. This makes harsh self-criticism seem less powerful and helps you see thoughts just as thoughts, not truths.

Activity 15.2: Values Mapping: Find What Matters

In this activity, write down what is truly important to you in life (values like kindness, honesty, growth, etc.).

____

____

____

____

When self-hatred shows up, remind yourself that you can choose actions—small or large—that align with your values, even if you feel upset or critical of yourself.

Activity 15.3: Acceptance Exercise: Make Space for Feelings

When self-hatred arises, pause and take three slow breaths. Silently say to yourself, "I notice this thought and this feeling," without trying to judge it or push it away. Imagine making space in your mind for those feelings as you would for a guest—they don't have to control your actions, and they are not permanent.

Part 5

Finding Hope and Technology's Limit

The purpose of *I Hate Myself* and this workbook is to bring you hope. Your future self can have a better daily life than your present self, and with some time and practice, you will get closer to becoming that future self. The activities in this section will help you prepare for long-term improvement. There are so many ways to ease your feelings of self-hatred that most people can gain relief using proven approaches like cognitive behavior therapy (CBT) and dialectical behavior therapy (DBT). Working with a skilled therapist is vitally important in helping you progress. Technology is not a substitute, so approach it with caution.

Part 5 Activity: Mirror Work

Having self-compassion means treating yourself with the same care and kindness that you would give to a friend. It gets easier with practice, and this activity is one way to do that. Consider your strengths, talents, and skills. Using the kindest language you can, write down five statements about yourself here. Use the second-person point of view (e.g., "You are a supportive friend.").

1. ______________________________

____

____

____

2. ____

____

____

____

3. ____

____

____

____

4. ____

____

____

____

5. ____

____

____

____

Now, take this list to a mirror and gradually make eye contact with yourself. While looking yourself in the eyes, repeat these statements sincerely and with self-compassion. Repeat this activity, progressing from neutral statements to kind statements. Accept your praise and believe it.

Chapter 16

Enduring Hope

Chapter Summary

One of the most important things to remember—and believe—about self-hatred is that you are not alone. People like you, who have experienced self-hatred, have been able to find self-compassion, break their negative thinking patterns, and improve the quality of their daily lives. Count yourself among them as you work with your therapist to find your own path to a you that reflects your true self rather than the flawed one that you were taught to believe was you.

Chapter 16 Warmup Activity: Embrace Enoughness

Let's begin this chapter with something a little different. Go online and watch Brené Brown's TED Talk about shame, "Gift of Imperfection." After you've finished it, answer the following question:

1. What would it look like to embrace "enoughness"?

____

____

____

____

Now, read the following paragraph and answer question 2.

The Impact of Social Media on Not Enoughness

Social media perpetuates self-hatred primarily by shaping distorted self-perceptions, reinforcing unattainable ideals, and exploiting human psychology's sensitivity to social comparison and validation. Modern digital ecosystems—driven by profit motives and algorithmic engagement—constantly target users' insecurities and condition self-worth to external approval. Social platforms prioritize highly curated, filtered, and idealized images—creating constant upward social comparisons. Users repeatedly compare themselves to digitally enhanced versions of others, leading to body dissatisfaction, inferiority, and shame. A 2025 study found that frequent social media users report lower self-esteem and increased depressive symptoms due to constant exposure to unrealistic success and beauty standards.

2. Reflect on the above paragraph and then consider the impact of social media on how you see yourself. Do you experience self-dissatisfaction or do you feel that a spotlight is shone on your self-hatred, making it hard to conclude anything other than that you are flawed?

   ____

   ____

   ____

   ____

Remember that, with practice, you will get better at the techniques in this book. It's important to work with your therapist to figure out what works best for you, and how you can overcome your feelings of self-hatred.

The Impact of Self-Hatred

This entire workbook is about tackling self-hatred, and as stated before, many of the exercises are variations of previous ones. The task each time is to continue to dig deeper into the questions and have more comprehensive, nuanced, and considered answers. If you have lived experience, you know more than anyone the impact of self-hatred and its profound negative impact on your mental, emotional, and physical well-being. It has likely influenced your self-esteem, relationships, behavior, and overall quality of life in multiple, and likely damaging, ways.

Here are some specific psychological and emotional impacts:

- **Low self-esteem and worthlessness:** Self-hatred undermines your self-worth, leading you to feel unlovable, defective, or inherently flawed, which can contribute to depression, anxiety, and hopelessness.
- **Increased risk of mental illness:** As you read in earlier chapters, self-hatred is closely tied to depression, anxiety disorders, eating disorders, and personality disorders, often exacerbating symptoms and complicating recovery.
- **Self-criticism and rumination:** Persistent negative self-talk fuels cycles of self-criticism and rumination, deepening emotional distress and reducing motivation for positive change, and reinforcing self-hatred.
- **Suicidal ideation and self-harm:** Extreme self-hatred increases your vulnerability to suicidal thoughts and self-injurious behaviors, which often function as a way to escape emotional pain or as a form of self-punishment. Again, suicide is not the answer.

There are also behavioral and social consequences:

- **Isolation and withdrawal:** You might avoid social interactions out of shame and fear of rejection, leading to loneliness and reduced support networks.
- **Impaired relationships:** Self-hatred impacts trust in others, intimacy, and communication, making relationships fraught with conflict or detachment.
- **Maladaptive coping:** Self-hatred may manifest as maladaptive coping behaviors, including substance use, procrastination, and neglect of self-care.

Fear of Getting Better

The final exercise that people with lived experience have said helps with self-hatred is tackling the fear of getting better. This seems like a paradox, and it is experienced as the anxiety or resistance you have toward recovery, healing, or improvement, even when you consciously desire to feel better. Here is why this happens:

- **First, there is the fear of the unknown:** Recovery involves change, and change can be unsettling or frightening, especially after long periods of self-hatred. The familiar, even if painful, feels safer than the unknown new normal.
- **Identity and self-definition:** For many people with self-hatred, the issue is core to their identity. Getting rid of it may feel like losing a core part of who you are, leading to confusion or fear about "who I will be" without self-hatred.
- **Fear of responsibility:** Having less self-hatred means that you have to participate more fully in life and with this it can feel as if you have new responsibilities for maintaining your wellbeing and making new life choices, which can feel overwhelming.
- **Fear of disappointment or failure:** If you struggle with self-hatred, and are dealing with it and making healthier choics, concerns about relapse or setbacks can make maintaining your recovery seem risky or discouraging for fear that you will disappoint yourself and others if you should fail.

For more on the fear of getting better, see Activity 16.1.

A note for therapists: *Use these worksheets to help clients experiment with new perspectives, challenge old narratives, and build self-compassion. Encourage clients to share their completed worksheets in session for discussion and support. Integrate these lived-experience strategies with DBT, ACT, CBT, and mindfulness skills as appropriate.*

Activity 16.1: Tackling the Fear of Getting Better

Explore your feelings about getting better, and focus on the emotions that might be a little uncomfortable. Now, answer the following questions:

- What fears come up when you imagine feeling better or recovering? In particular, what would it feel like to be a you who does not hate yourself? List all of your fears.

  ____

  ____

  ____

  ____

- How does shame or fear of change keep you stuck?

  ____

  ____

  ____

  ____

- Are you worried that people will now start to think that you are all better and have more demands of you?

  ____

  ____

  ____

  ____

- What is one fear, even if small, that you can address in the next week?

  ____

  ____

  ____

  ____

Activity 16.2: Who Are You Beyond Self-Hatred?

Consider yourself as a person who, while you might have some flaws, also has some incredible strengths. See yourself as a whole person, focusing beyond the flaws but also on your best attributes. What are these more positive qualities? If you need help, talk to someone who cares for you to get ideas. Now answer the following questions:

List your values, strengths, or roles. Here are some positive core values: integrity, compassion, respect, responsibility, honesty, fairness, courage, generosity, gratitude, perseverance, and accountability. Write "I have integrity," "I am compassionate," "I am respectful," etc.

____

____

____

____

What is one thing you can do to better align with a value (e.g., creativity → doodle for five minutes; a good listener → call a friend who might need a listener).

____

____

____

____

Activity 16.3: Behavioral Change (DBT and CBT)

Every emotion that we have triggers action urges: Anger drives attack, fear drives avoidance, sadness drives withdrawal, and shame drives hiding. Opposite action is a DBT skill that disrupts these automatic responses by encouraging behavior that contradicts the urge—thereby reshaping both emotion and your body's reaction. In other words, changing your behavior will change your brain and its responses. Self-hatred is fueled by shame, self-punishment, and chronic avoidance of self-acceptance. By behaving as if your self is worthy of dignity and care, emotions begin to follow behavior. For example, maintaining your hygiene, wearing clothes that express individuality, or sharing opinions assertively—even when self-loathing urges you to do the opposite—you can slowly retrain emotional circuits toward neutrality and eventual self-respect.

Many who struggle with self-hatred engage in behaviors that appear to validate negative beliefs, including that they are deserving of punishment. Opposite action targets this by introducing deliberate self-compassion actions—resting when tired, accepting compliments, or acknowledging small successes—thus breaking reinforcement cycles of guilt and punishment.

1. What is one self-punishing behavior (e.g., skipping meals, overworking) that you engage in?

   ____

   ____

   ____

   ____

2. How can you commit to making a small behavioral change by doing something opposite to a behavior that keeps you stuck in self-hatred?

   ____

   ____

   ____

   ____

3. Consider how you can further practice "opposite action" (e.g., eat a nourishing meal despite feeling "undeserving") to change your behavior? What opposite action can you take today?

   ____

   ____

   ____

   ____

Activity 16.4: Self-Compassion Toolkit

This activity is designed to help prevent relapses. While it's normal to slip up now and again, it can be helpful to have a crisis plan in case you feel overwhelmed. Answer the following questions to put together your crisis plan.

1. Choose a calming mantra ("This is my shame talking, it is not my truth"). Write it down here.

____

____

____

____

2. Identify a go-to self-care action (e.g., shower, walk in nature).

____

____

____

____

3. Create a list of people you find praiseworthy, including what you admire about each of them. Would you want your future self to be similar to the admired people and want to have their attributes?

____

____

____

____

Activity 16.5: Externalize the Critic (IFS)

You have learned about many different types of therapy: DBT, CBT, EMDR and so on. Here is a new one: internal family systems (IFS). IFS sees the mind as made up of "parts," including the inner critic, the achiever, the pleaser, etc. organized around a core Self that is naturally calm, compassionate, and capable of leading the system. In IFS, the goal is not to get rid of parts, but to help the Self build a trusting relationship with them so their roles can become less extreme and more helpful. The Self is seen as the central, undamaged core characterized by qualities often called the eight C's: calm, curiosity, clarity, compassion, confidence, courage, creativity, and connectedness.

Externalizing the critic is a therapeutic technique from IFS where you learn to see your internal self-critical voice—the "inner critic"—as a separate entity rather than a fundamental part of who you are. This approach is particularly powerful in addressing self-hatred because it creates psychological distance from harsh self-judgments and allows for more objective evaluation and compassionate interaction with these thoughts.

1. Self-hatred is often fueled by an internalized voice that attacks your worth and identity. By externalizing this critical voice—giving it a name, an image, or a persona—you can recognize that these harsh judgments are not inherently "you" but rather learned messages or maladaptive parts trying to protect them or express unmet needs. Write down what your inner critic is regularly telling you.

   ____

   ____

   ____

   ____

View this voice as something external to you, engage with it as you would with another person: question its motives, set boundaries, or even challenge its accuracy. This will foster empowerment and agency and diminish your feelings of helplessness associated with the voice of self-hatred.

2. Externalizing allows you the space to uncover why your critic is so vocal—often rooted in past trauma, fear, or internalized and negative societal messages from your youth. Recognizing these origins enables cultivating compassion toward oneself and the critic. This compassionate stance reduces the intensity of self-hate and promotes healing. Is there any person or people from your past who sound exactly like your critic? Who are they and what did they say?

   ____

   ____

   ____

   ____

A Step-by-Step Guide to **Externalizing the Inner Critic**

The basic idea is: separate from it, see it as a part, then relate to it from Self rather than fusing with it.

1. Name and notice it as a part
    - When you hear self-attacking thoughts, label them: "A critical part is here," rather than "I am terrible."
    - You might give it a nickname (e.g., "The Taskmaster" or "The Perfectionist") to reinforce that it is a part of you, not the whole you.
2. Give it an image and location
    - Let yourself sense: If this critic had an age, posture, or outfit, what would it look like? Where is it in or around your body?
    - Visualizing it as a distinct figure (e.g., a stern teacher, anxious parent, or scared teenager) helps externalize and create internal space.
3. Access Self and adjust distance
    - Notice your own reaction to the critic (annoyed, scared, ashamed) and ask those reacting parts to "step back a little" so more calm curiosity can be present.
    - From that more Self-led place (calmer, more compassionate), imagine sitting across from the critic, as if in a room or at a table, so you can talk *with* it instead of *from* it.
4. Start a respectful dialogue
    - Ask the critic questions like: "What are you afraid would happen if you didn't talk to me this way?" or "How long have you been doing this job?"
    - Listen for its fears (e.g., "You'll be rejected," "You'll repeat an old humiliation") and reflect back understanding, without arguing or trying to silence it.
5. Appreciate intention, renegotiate strategy
    - Explicitly acknowledge that it has been working hard to protect you, even if its methods hurt: this appreciation often reduces its intensity.
    - From Self, explore alternatives: ask if it would be open to trying a different role (e.g., encouraging coach, discerning advisor) once the underlying vulnerable parts (exiles) get more care.

6. Return to the exiles it protects
   - As trust builds, the critic will often reveal memories or younger feelings it is guarding; these are typically the exiles carrying shame, fear, or grief.
   - In IFS therapy, the work then shifts toward helping Self connect directly with those exiles so they can release burdens, which in turn allows the critic to relax its extreme stance.

Key Points

- Social media perpetuate self-hatred by creating constant upward comparisons that can lead to feelings of inadequacy.
- Self-hatred profoundly impacts mental health (depression, anxiety, suicidal ideation), relationships (isolation, impaired trust), and behaviors (maladaptive coping, self-harm).
- Fear of getting better is real, and recovery brings unknown changes, identity shifts, new responsibilities, and risk of disappointment or relapse.
- Opposite action (behaving as if you're worthy despite self-hatred urges) gradually retrains emotional circuits toward self-respect and breaks punishment cycles.

Chapter 17

AI's Take on Self-Hatred

Chapter Summary

This final chapter is somewhat irreverent because it was the one section where I used artificial intelligence (AI). I used AI to make a case against itself, and so the reader might smile at the absurdity of the exercise. Remember that AI is a powerful tool that has recently been applied to nearly every industry on the planet, including therapy. Despite the tremendous interest in this technological tool, it's important that people are cautious about using AI as a mental health treatment or a substitute for a therapist. Based on my interactions with AI, it continues to come across as non-human. It lacks empathy and understanding, and provides predictable and very variable suggestions. Remember that an AI tool is *not* a person, so it cannot relate to humans, understand the human experience, or connect on an emotional level with sincerity.

I asked Perplexity, an AI tool, why AI is so unempathetic, and this is what it answered:

> *AI systems like mine come across as non-human and lacking in empathy because they do not possess consciousness, feelings, or lived experience. Instead, they generate responses by processing vast amounts of text data and identifying patterns—relying on algorithms to predict what words or phrases are most likely to follow a given prompt, rather than truly understanding or "feeling" anything.*

As humans, we thrive on human connection, and although AI systems can solve complex computational problems and entertain us at times, they will never truly connect in a way that people with conditions like self-hatred truly need.

AI Answers Why *Not* to Use AI!

I asked Perplexity to tell me why I should not use AI to help address self-hatred (accessed October 14, 2025, on perplexity.ai). The answers say it all!

Why AI Seems Non-Human

- AI does not have a mind, self-awareness, or subjective experience—it processes information, but does not feel or think like humans do.
- Its language may imitate empathy, but the underlying mechanism is pattern-matching, not emotional resonance or intuitive understanding.
- AI lacks body language, tone, and real-time emotional context, making its responses sometimes appear robotic, too formal, or stereotyped.

Why AI Lacks Empathy

- Empathy in humans involves both feeling (emotional empathy) and understanding (cognitive empathy) what another person is experiencing, often based on personal history and social learning.
- AI can simulate empathetic language, but this is imitation—a statistical generation of words that "sound" empathetic based on examples in its training data, not genuine emotional concern.
- AI cannot "care" in the way humans do; it has no internal motivation, no sense of relationship, and no nervous system that responds to another's distress.

Limits and Advances

While developers continually improve AI's ability to recognize emotional cues and generate more supportive or sensitive responses, they cannot give AI real empathy or a true sense of connection—current systems only mimic these qualities by statistical association, not inner experience.

This means that, although AI tools can be useful for information, coaching, or reminders, they'll always feel non-human and fundamentally different from genuine, compassionate human interaction.

In Conclusion

AIs like these should not be used as a primary tool for tackling self-hatred because it fundamentally lacks the empathy, lived experience, and nuanced judgment that are essential in deep psychological healing. While AI can offer supportive information and coping strategies, there are several critical limitations for addressing complex issues like self-hatred:

Lack of Genuine Empathy and Human Connection

- AI can mimic empathetic language but doesn't feel compassion or form authentic, reciprocal relationships—key ingredients for recovering from self-hatred and developing self-worth.
- Genuine healing often arises from feeling deeply understood by another person, something AI simply cannot provide.

Risk of Reinforcing Harmful Patterns

- AI may inadvertently validate negative self-beliefs if it lacks context or misinterprets user input, potentially reinforcing self-hatred or giving unsafe advice.
- Without specialized oversight, users can become overly reliant on AI for validation or emotional support, leading to isolation or addiction to technology rather than fostering real-world resilience and relationships.

Absence of Complex Clinical Judgment

- Skilled therapists use intuition, clinical experience, and subtle social cues to adapt care for unique patient histories and situations. AI systems cannot personalize support in the way a human therapist can.
- AI cannot recognize nonverbal distress, assess risk accurately, or intervene in emergencies as safely as a trained clinician.

Ethical and Safety Concerns

- There is a risk of unethical guidance, breaches of confidentiality, or exposure to harmful concepts if AI systems are used without appropriate human oversight, especially for vulnerable individuals struggling with profound self-hatred.

Key Points

- AI lacks genuine empathy, consciousness, and lived experience—it only mimics compassion through pattern-matching, not true emotional understanding.
- AI cannot form authentic relationships or provide the human connection essential for healing from self-hatred.
- Risks of using AI for self-hatred include reinforcing harmful patterns, overreliance on technology, inability to assess safety/risk, and potential for unethical guidance.
- AI lacks clinical judgment, cannot read nonverbal cues, and cannot adapt care with the nuance and intuition of trained human therapists.
- While AI can provide information and reminders, it should never replace genuine therapeutic relationships for addressing complex emotional issues like self-hatred.

Conclusion

As you close this workbook, remember that self-hatred is not a life sentence but a distortion that your mind has created, and one that you have the strength to overcome. Each step you take—no matter how small—can be a powerful act of courage and self-compassion. This journey is not about perfection but about embracing your humanity with kindness, curiosity, and hope. In having worked through this book, you and your therapist have laid the foundation for enduring change, resilience, and a future where self-acceptance grows stronger every day. Believe in your capacity to rewrite your story and move toward a life filled with dignity, purpose, and peace—you are not alone, and a much kinder you to yourself is possible.

Acknowledgments

I would like to acknowledge my team at Wiley, and in particular, Leah Zarra and Gabriela Mancuso. Then, to my excellent editor, Christina Verigan, who made this project much easier than I could have imagined. Then to my social media manager and dear friend KP. Finally, to Dax Shepard and Monica Padman, as well as all the other incredible podcasters who made *IHMS* such a success!

About the Author

Blaise Aguirre, MD, is a child and adolescent psychiatrist and an assistant professor of psychiatry at Harvard Medical School. He is a trainer in and specializes in dialectical behavior therapy (DBT) as well as other treatments for borderline personality disorder and associated conditions. He is the founding medical director of 3East continuum of care, an array of programs for teens and young adults that use DBT to target the symptoms of borderline personality disorder (BPD) and related conditions.

Dr. Aguirre has been a staff psychiatrist at McLean Hospital since 2000 and is nationally and internationally recognized for his extensive work in the treatment of mood and personality disorders in adolescents. He lectures regularly throughout the world. Dr. Aguirre is the author or co-author of multiple books, including *I Hate Myself, Borderline Personality Disorder in Adolescents, Mindfulness for Borderline Personality Disorder, Coping With BPD,* and the best-selling *DBT For Dummies.*

Index